Life in the Fast Lane

The Chris Stoddart Story

by Chris Stoddart

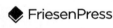 FriesenPress

One Printers Way
Altona, MB R0G 0B0
Canada

www.friesenpress.com

Copyright © 2022 by Chris Stoddart
First Edition — 2022

While every effort was made to ensure the information enclosed was correct, information from the early years of wheelchair sports was difficult at times and there may be instances where there is an incorrection.

All rights reserved.

No part of this publication may be reproduced in any form, or by any means, electronic or mechanical, including photocopying, recording, or any information browsing, storage, or retrieval system, without permission in writing from FriesenPress.

ISBN
978-1-03-914651-8 (Hardcover)
978-1-03-914650-1 (Paperback)
978-1-03-914652-5 (eBook)

1. BIOGRAPHY & AUTOBIOGRAPHY, SPORTS

Distributed to the trade by The Ingram Book Company

Table of Contents

Prologue: The Phone Call	ix
Chapter 1: Wheelchair Sports	1
Chapter 2: Let the Games Begin	13
Chapter 3: One Step Forward – One Step Back	38
Chapter 4: A Taste of Success	43
Chapter 5: Starting Over	49
Chapter 6: First Step Up	53
Chapter 7: Redemption	69
Chapter 8: Overcoming Obstacles	82
Chapter 9: Calm Before the Storm	107
Chapter 10: House of Cards	109
Chapter 11: Year of The Disabled	120
Chapter 12: Penalty Free	130
Chapter 13: A Job for Life	142
Chapter 14: Silver Lining	150
Chapter 15: A Year to Remember	166
Chapter 16: A New Ride	177
Chapter 17: Reaching for The Top	188
Chapter 18: Show's Over	205
Chapter 19: Change of Pace	219
Chapter 20: Three-Wheelers	225
Chapter 21: On the Road	230
Post-Script	233

To My Amazing Parents, Jack & Dot Stoddart…
Who Loved Me Enough To Let Me Try Anything

To My Big Brother Dave…
Who Has Always Been There For Me

To My Wonderful Wife Bev…
Who Brought Me Out Of The Darkness And
Keeps Me In The Light

Prologue: The Phone Call

Growing up with a disability, in my case, spina bifida, it meant overcoming obstacles was just a way of life, and when I entered high school, I had to decide what I wanted to do for a living once I graduated.

While growing up in the small village of Arthur Ontario, for as long as I can remember I wanted to be a radio announcer. As a kid, it began with Foster Hewitt, who's descriptions of games involving my beloved Toronto Maple Leafs kept me glued to the radio, and later to our television set. As I grew older, it was his son, Bill Hewitt that I listened to avidly. I still have the autographed picture he sent me when I was ten years old.

But as I became a teenager in the early 60's, rock and roll took hold of me. And as much as I loved hockey, I realized I loved music more, and one day my idol became a voice on the radio that lived for rock and roll and howled at the moon as well. American disc jockey, the iconic Wolfman Jack, spoke to me. This was something I could do, and I didn't need legs to get it done. From that day forward I dreamed of the day I would have my own radio show.

After graduating from Arthur District High School in the summer of '69, I set my sights on one of the Communication Programs at Ryerson University in Toronto. When they wouldn't take me over concerns that my wheelchair would not be able to navigate around the floor cameras, or into the control booths, I reset my sights and turned my attention to the new Seneca College in Scarborough.

So back in the Fall of '71, I was going to school like thousands of other young men in Canada. And in my case, getting through my third semester of Applied Communications.

Through a federal program for the disabled, I received funding to go to college and live in Toronto. The program also enabled me to lease a vehicle to get back and forth to classes, up to my parent's cottage in Buckhorn, or back to Arthur to see my girlfriend and/or my buddies. At the time of the phone call, I was quite happy in the basement of a house in North York. Bill McKee and his mom lived near Newtonbrook High School where Bill was enrolled, and it was an easy drive for me to reach Markham and Finch where the college was located.

One night during the week, we were hanging out in the living-room, listening to records on his mom's stereo when the phone rang. It was my big brother Dave. He was reading an article in the Toronto Star about wheelchair basketball. There were a group of guys in wheelchairs, who were looking for more players so that they could form a team and join an organization called the National Wheelchair Basketball Association (NWBA), that had dozens and dozens of wheelchair basketball teams scattered throughout the US. The Vancouver Cable Cars were the only Canadian entry, and these guys were trying to become the second.

When I got off the phone, I called the manager Bev Hallam, and he gave me the time and directions to the gym. I had no idea how much my life would be forever changed.

Chapter 1: Wheelchair Sports

Perhaps it was Fate behind that first phone call, since I have always loved to go fast. I think someone must have left the side of my crib down one day, and I spied freedom. Once I learned to crawl, I was on my way, and there was no turning back. I was a crawling machine. As small as I was back then, I got a lot of strange looks though as I scrambled across the lawns of my Etobicoke neighbours. Considering my size and weight, I guess it was no wonder my first childhood nickname, bestowed upon me during my first year in public school was *Spider*.

Naturally, being born with a disability, there was no "Ah Ha" or "Uh Oh" moment when I realized something bad had happened. I can't say I was in the middle of crawling somewhere when I suddenly started thinking, "What's wrong with this picture?"

In kindergarten, and after a few operations to "straighten things out" so to speak, I found myself up on wooden crutches, learning to balance on long leg braces. At about 3 feet standing upright, the air up there was quite rarified! "You can see a lot farther from up here", I thought to myself. But it was the only advantage.

I was painfully slow. I had to brace my arms on my crutches and swing my legs through, balance, and then move the crutches forward. Repeat after me... I can remember it used to drive me crazy, and every chance I got, I ditched the braces and crutches, and crawled like a bug on Ritalin to where I needed to go. Stares came with the territory, but a guy has to get there somehow. Take a picture. Tell your friends. There's a *Spider* on the loose.

A couple of years later, and after another operation, I was fitted with a new set of braces, along with a pair of new-fangled aluminum crutches that fit on your forearms, instead of under your arms like I was used to. They were necessary if I was going to learn to walk a "more normal" way, but I was even slower and felt more ungainly than ever. Swing one leg forward, move the opposite side crutch forward. Other leg forward, opposite crutch forward. Repeat, repeat, repeat. Looking back, it makes me laugh now, because it reminds me of going to the racetrack to watch the trotters in action… in slow motion.

I got better over time, but I ditched them every chance I could. On my little street called Rathburn Road in Etobicoke, no-one seemed to mind, but when I found myself in Grade Two in a different public school, I realized the practise was not as well received, shall we say. No place to crawl and when I did, it evoked a reaction that I was not expecting. Political correctness had yet to be invented, and so my *Spider* nickname was replaced with *Chris Cripple* or variations along that line.

I was miserable at school, and it was only a year or so later that Dad sat me down and said we were moving out of the city and going to a small place called Arthur. Over the years, reporters would always ask, "Port Arthur?" No, just Arthur. North of Orangeville, at the crossroads of Highways 6 and 9.

Strangest thing about Arthur though. It was like I had entered the Twilight Zone. The town seemed like a bigger version of Rathburn Rd. I just blended in. No-one blinked an eye.

My parent bought a grocery store called the Red & White, situated on Main Street, and we lived in the 3-bedroom apartment above. Soon I was enrolled in Arthur Public School, population: not that many. Kids from town and the rest bussed in from all the farms and the smaller surrounding communities.

On the second day in town, I met a kid named Keith Colwill. I was working my way down the street on my crutches, when he came up to me and asked me what had happened. I explained my situation and he said something like, "Oh too bad". I told him that my parents had bought the grocery store, and it turned out his family lived almost directly behind us on the next street. When I mentioned I had a pet turtle, he came over to see and our friendship was sealed forever.

Chapter 1: Wheelchair Sports

We were best friends from that day forward, and even though he is a retired RCMP officer living in BC, and we don't get a chance to see each other very much, I will be eternally grateful for his friendship growing up in Arthur. He cast a big shadow and starting from day one in public school and all through high school, if anyone had visions of giving me a hard time, he was there if need be. He never had to fight on my behalf though, his presence was more than enough to discourage anyone interested in pressing the point. No wonder he became a great Mountie.

Compared to the city, going to school in the country was a dream come true. Lots of room to run around and play. Or in my case, crawl around and play. Which never raised an eyebrow. Everyone just bought into the idea that crawling was my preferred way of getting around. I got in the habit of slowly walking to school, ditching my crutches under my desk, and crawling around for the rest of the day. Outside at recess or up the hall to the washroom. It was all good.

Soon I was learning to play catch, sitting on the ground and throwing a softball back and forth to Keith or one of my other school mates. I learned to dive sideways for the ones my buddies threw off-line, but they got accurate real fast. I only sat about two feet off the ground, and if you sailed it over my head, you were the one that had to go retrieve it!

I liked playing soccer at recess as well, using my hands to move the ball along or pass to a teammate. By Grade 6, I was still fast enough on the ground to keep up playing with the guys, but one day it all ended rather suddenly.

We usually had a lively game of soccer going on during lunch, and one day there was a loose ball, and I was crawling as fast as I could to get there before anyone else did. I went to hit the ball with my hand at the same time my school mate Phillip Green attempted to kick the ball with his foot. Too bad. We both missed the ball and he kicked me in the head instead.

They say he picked me up and ran into the classroom, me all limp and whatnot, and it wasn't until I woke up and found myself stretched out on my teacher's desk, that I realized what had happened. Naturally, the Principal, Mr. Cherry, was suitably freaked out, and for the rest of my time at Arthur Public, I was official scorekeeper or referee. But once school was out, I was free to do whatever.

Fast forward a few years, and after a month or so into Grade 9, I found myself back in the hospital for another operation and combined with a 6-month stay rehabbing at the Crippled Children's Centre in Toronto, (now the Hugh McMillan Centre), it meant I missed a lot of school and just barely moved on.

During my time off school though, I came to realize a few things. First off, I realized that going to high school presented new challenges. Though I still crawled around in gym class, I used my crutches the rest of the time, but being so small, I got knocked over all the time in the rush of my fellow classmates on their way from class to class. Not on purpose, but considering I still only came up to everyone's chest and I weighed a massive 65 lbs, it was no wonder I found myself down and out a few times a day.

Secondly, while I was off school, I began looking at girls a lot differently and realized that hitting the floor every day was decidedly uncool. I needed to be more mobile.

My ultimate course of action occurred to me during my last visit to the doctor's office, as he explained what he had in store for me next. I asked him how many more operations would be needed before I was walking normally. I guess, even as a young teenager, I still didn't grasp the extent of my disability and I was looking for "some kind of miracle" that would make me normal.

When he explained that I would never walk without crutches and braces, I politely told him, and my parents, that there would be no more operations. I had decided otherwise. At that point in my life, I realized I needed to go in another direction. I wanted a wheelchair.

Getting a chair of my own had been a secret goal of mine ever since I went to Crippled Children's Camp for the first time.

A few years after we had moved to Arthur, my parents announced that I was going to Lakewood, a crippled children's camp for three weeks. A camp full of disabled kids? I had my doubts. Frankly, I was not all that thrilled. We were already out in the country where I could go fishing whenever I wanted to. I didn't really want to go, but naturally I had no choice.

But, once at camp, I found that there were lots of extra wheelchairs to use, and my favourite became a small *Johnson & Johnson* wheelchair that I could fly in. With all the paved pathways that weaved in and around the camp, I could motor around for hours for the pure joy of going fast. I had

Chapter 1: Wheelchair Sports

three weeks of cruising around and I only used my crutches when I had to. Every year for the four years I went there in the summer, I ditched the crutches and went wheeling.

It wasn't long before I had become friends with a bunch of the guys and since the camp had paved trails all over the facility, we could wheel for miles without going off camp property. I loved the freedom that the wheelchair provided. I hoped I'd have one of my own some day.

But, since my parents picked out my wheelchair, I didn't end up with a small J & J "hot rod" that I raced around at Lakewood. Instead, this chair was like a four-door Cadillac. All chrome, but massive. I could carry three books on either side of me, and in high school pictures from back then, I looked like Lily Tomlin's *Edith Ann* character from the old '70's Laugh-In television show. Didn't matter though. My world got a lot easier, and I felt so much better than walking around like the Tin Man from the Wizard of Oz.

During the summer I wheeled back and forth to school with my buddies from town, but once snow arrived, I needed a ride. Arthur is smack dab in the middle of the snowbelt, and we had snowstorms growing up back then that pales anything I have been through since. Sometimes the whole town was snowed in, literally for days. And since my parents were busy running the store, it meant they took me to school early or I stayed home.

Dad's solution was a new-fangled machine called a snowmobile. Ours was called a Rustler. It went about 50 mph, which was fast for the 60's. It made for great high-speed runs down the back streets of town, and I was always available if one of the gals wanted a quick ride home at lunch or wanted to go for a ride after school before the busses arrived to pick up the out-of-towners. My buddies would turn the machine around for me and I kept my wheelchair near the front door, since I crawled around at home most of the time.

It was fun for a year or so, but eventually the guys started getting their driver's licenses and I was becoming a perpetual passenger. I wished I could get my license, even though the guys always found a spot for me and my date in the back seat. And that's not a bad thing.

I'm not sure how my Dad found out about hand controls for cars, but one day at the kitchen table, he showed me an article with a car that had been equipped with them. He said it was about time I started fending for myself. Although the new car we were getting was for Mom, I would be able to use it to get back and forth to school. But of course, it was not long before "going to school" became "see you later", and I had wheels of my own.

Dad sent away to British Columbia for the hand controls and one of the local garages in town installed them in our new car, a blue 4-door 1968 Buick Special.

Wheelchairs back then were heavy and cumbersome. No super light titanium frames, no popping your wheels off with quick release axles or chairbacks that folded down, like we have now. I got in the habit of climbing in the back seat on the driver's side, folding my chair behind the front bench seat, hopping over the seat, and I was good to go. In the beginning I would sit on my legs for added height, but eventually I used a cushion.

Once I wrote my learner's test and got my temporary license, another high school buddy, Craig Mulholland taught me how to drive around town. Dad made an appointment for me to take my test in Mount Forest, a small-town north of us, but it was in three months. I managed to get an appointment in Guelph that was only three weeks away. Dad said fine, but if I flunked, I would have to take Driver's Ed when school started. No problem. No worries.

How was I to know Guelph had multiple stoplights, going which-way and whatnot, and after a couple of not seeing the correct stoplight, I flunked the test.

Dad laughed because he knew I didn't want to have to take lessons like the kids that "couldn't get the hang of it on their own", but as luck would have it, a couple of weeks after I flunked the first one, the Mount Forest office called and said they had an opening. Off I went.

The day of the test had Craig and I sitting there in the waiting room, biding our time until my number was called. And when it was, I looked up to see the same instructor who had flunked me in Guelph. He smiled and said, "Are you trying to get away from me?" I nervously said no, but he was just having a bit of fun.

And as luck would have it, Mount Forest only had one stoplight and I did not run it, so we cruised back to Arthur with my first license and full of excitement. That car served me well for the last couple of years of high school and Mom got it back when I headed to college.

As promised, I showed up on time to the high school gym that was situated in downtown Toronto where the team practised. Wheeling in, I began to watch these guys roll up and down the court, doing lay-ups, dribbling with one hand, pushing the chair with the other hand, and shooting baskets from around the key. I was quite impressed.

It wasn't long before the manager saw me and rolled over to introduce himself. Though a quadriplegic by virtue of an accident when he was younger, Bev nonetheless motored around in his electric chair with unbridled determination. In the years to follow, he never ceased to amaze me with his drive and the amount of work he accomplished in expanding wheelchair sports in Ontario and Canada. He was a founding member of the group that formed the Canadian Wheelchair Sports Association (CWSA) back in 1967.

He brought me over to introduce me to all the guys, and while most of them were friendly, a couple of them wasted no time in giving me the gears. Billy Brouse was a big guy, but his buddy Brian Halliday, was nothing short of huge. I had never seen someone in a wheelchair that was so muscular. He looked like a weightlifter, and later in the evening I would find out that he was just that.

First thing Brian said to me was, "Who the hell are you supposed to be?" I guess my being a 4-foot six-inch 80 lb weakling, with shoulder length hair and wearing a studded black leather jacket, sitting in what they thought was a gold-coloured wheelchair, struck them as funny! But after a closer inspection, Billy pointed out that the chair was really all rust, not gold colored, which made them laugh even harder. As I was thinking to myself that I might have made a mistake here, I realized they were just goofing with me. It was the beginning of a life-long friendship with the two of them as we would spend more than a decade of travelling together as teammates.

The Toronto Thunderbolt's coach was Gord Paterson, winner of the gold medal in the 60 metres at the '68 Paralympics, and like Bev, he contributed to the formation of the C.W.S.A. Looking back, he reminds me a lot of Pat Burns, the late great coach of the Toronto Maple Leafs. Neither suffered fools lightly. Gord was all business and expected your undivided attention when he was talking and a full effort during the drills and games. Watching him bounce the ball off a teammate's face when Coach caught him staring off into space while he was talking, ensured that I always paid close attention. I had already managed to get my nose broken twice and I didn't think a third time would be lucky.

Not long after practise began, it was apparent that I had more speed in my old rust-bucket than anyone expected. Turned out I was fast. Not super fast but Coach was pleased. The team needed someone to run the fast break and who could shoot as well.

Now I shot hoops with my buddies all through high school, and I worked the scoreboard for both the boys' and girls' school league games, so I did know the basics of basketball. As well at the time, one of our neighbours up in Buckhorn was the late Al Waters of CHUM 1050 radio fame. They had a cottage just up the road from us, complete with a tennis court and basketball net. On the weekends, when we were not out fishing, or I wasn't driving the boat so he could waterski with his friends, Dave and I would shoot hoops.

I didn't have much strength back then and I couldn't get the ball high enough to get it in the basket using the proper shooting technique and so I would just kind of use a one-handed shot-put motion to get the height I needed. In the sixteen years I ended up playing basketball, my technique didn't improve much, but I did learn to perfect my one-hand shot, so eventually I was able to be accurate while on the move or hiding behind a screen for an outside shot.

One of the other guys on the team, by the name of Bob Simpson, was lightning fast on the court and the other quick guy looked familiar, but I couldn't figure out where I had seen him. Billy said his name was Mike O'Brien, and that he kept to himself, but the name didn't ring a bell. It would take a while before I figured where I had seen him.

As practise progressed, I realized that I did have an advantage over Bob and Mike, for while they were faster than me in their chairs, they couldn't shoot the basketball as well as I could, despite my poor technique. Besides, Bob was heavily into wheelchair racing.

Wheelchair racing? That was an even bigger surprise than the existence of wheelchair basketball. Earlier in practise, I had mentioned to Brian that

Chapter 1: Wheelchair Sports

Bob was sure quick in his chair, and that's when he told me Bob was the fastest man in the world in a wheelchair.

How did he know that? Wheelchair sports. Track, field events, swimming, weightlifting. All kinds of events. Provincial games, national championships, world championships, and the ultimate of all sports, our own Olympics. Or Paralympics as they would eventually be known as.

Bob held the world record in his disability class for the 100 metres at 19 seconds. And when I got talking with Bob after practise, he thought that with some work, I might be able to challenge a guy named Frank Henderson of New Brunswick, who was the reigning Canadian track champion in what they thought would be my disability class. I was lost for words.

The guys told me something else important, in that all these competitions were made possible through the efforts of hundreds of volunteers in all the provinces and countries that had a disabled sports program. And that money was scarce in the world of disabled sports, so if I wanted to make the Ontario team I had to compete in as many events as possible. The next day I called my brother and told him all about wheelchair sports.

The origins of wheelchair competitions can be traced back to the post-Second World War rehabilitation efforts at a hospital in Aylesbury England called Stoke Mandeville. They started through the efforts of Dr (and eventually) Sir Ludwig Guttman, who was and still is, considered to be the father of wheelchair sports. It was Dr. Guttman who realized that sport could help motivate disabled veterans into overcoming their loss of self-esteem and at the same time show others that, even though a person was disabled, there was no reason for that to prevent them from working and enjoying life. And being fit and as healthy as possible helped extend the life of those confined to a wheelchair.

From those modest beginnings, disabled games matured to become excellent athletic events, evolving from a rehabilitation level to a level of true sporting competition.

The first organized competition at Stoke Mandeville was among the hospital's patients, and took place on July 28th, 1948, and eventually, by 1952 they had expanded internationally. The competitions were now called the

Stoke Mandeville Games. In that first year, the games were contested by over a hundred athletes from Great Britain and the Netherlands.

Canada's first involvement in wheelchair competition was a recorded athletic event involving wheelchair athletes in 1947 at the Deer Lodge Rehabilitation Hospital in Winnipeg, although Canada did not enter a team in the first Paralympics that had been held in Rome, Italy in 1960.

We were also absent at the 1964 Games, held in Tokyo, Japan. However, fortunately for us, a doctor who worked with our Olympic team wondered why Canada was not represented. After talking with Dr. Guttman, they formulated a plan to get Canada into international competition.

Doctor Robert W. Jackson went back to Canada determined to ensure we had a team for the next games, and all these years later, and even though he has passed on, our "Father of Disabled Sports" is still admired for all the work he did in making Canada, not just participants, but an eventual world power and a strong voice in the development of disabled sports worldwide.

The first interprovincial competition among Canadian disabled athletes was held in the summer of 1967 in Montreal, and later in the year, through the efforts of many, the first ever Pan-American Wheelchair Games were held in Winnipeg, with athletes from Argentina, Jamaica, Mexico, Trinidad and Tobago, Canada and the United States competing.

The success of these games helped tremendously as Dr. Jackson had already begun to gather all the interested disabled clubs that had sprung up throughout Canada together, and on September 9th of that same year the Canadian Wheelchair Sports Association was formed with 7 of the 10 Provinces represented. Dr. Jackson and Toronto Thunderbolt Manager Bev Hallam represented Ontario on that first Board.

America entered a team in the first Paralympics and while they competed as a nation in all the events offered, wheelchair basketball seemed to be the sport that a great deal of US post-World War II veterans gravitated towards. Playing together as a team appealed to many of the young wounded, who wanted to get on with their lives. Basketball was their first love.

The Paralyzed Veterans of America was formed in 1946, and VA hospital teams began to form on both American coasts, as more and more disabled individuals discovered the excitement and friendship that wheelchair basketball provided.

Chapter 1: Wheelchair Sports

Originally, teams could only field paraplegics, but eventually the more inclusive National Wheelchair Basketball Association was formed, which allowed amputees, polio victims, and other disabled individuals to play wheelchair basketball. This was the league we were hoping to join.

As much as sports offered veterans and other individuals who were disabled later in life, an outlet, the untold number of people around the world, like me, who were born with some sort of disability that prevent them from ever testing their skills against their peers, were suddenly afforded the opportunity. I would venture to say that if games for the disabled had been restricted to only paraplegics, the phenomenal growth that disabled sports has enjoyed around the world over the decades, would not have reached the levels that the sport attained.

At the end of the following week's practise, Billy and I were over at Brian's parents' place planning for the upcoming summer. Bob had already invited me to train with him and Billy on the McMaster University track in Hamilton on the weekends once spring arrived, but being mindful that I had to be versatile, Billy suggested I also come to Hamilton and try swimming at the downtown YWCA where his swim coach, Corrie Steenkist, trained her disabled swimmers. I learned to swim at Lakewood Camp as a kid, but I didn't fancy myself quick by any stretch of the imagination, nor could I go far. But if it would help me get picked for the team, I would pretty much try anything.

As well, Brian suggested we get together in the spring and start throwing the discus and the shot putt. Seriously, the shot putt? But he kept reminding me that the more events I was entered in, the better chance I'd have of getting picked for the 1972 Calgary National Wheelchair Games scheduled for the following summer at the University of Alberta.

So, the next Saturday found me in downtown Hamilton, freezing my butt off while trying to do laps in the YWCA pool. Since Coach Corrie already had a stable of disabled swimmers under her wing, she had a good idea what class I would be in, but I would have to wait to be examined by the sport doctors in Guelph during classification at our Provincial Wheelchair Games in May before I would know for sure.

In the pool, sprinting seemed to be the way to go as far as my swimming events went. Coach said I was quick, but I burned out fast. The 50-metre freestyle, 50-metre backstroke, and the 50-metre breaststroke were fine. I tried the 75-metre medley as well, but any farther and I was heading for the bottom.

One of the great things about swimming with Coach Corrie's group, was being introduced to swimmer Hilda Binns. Not only did Hilda swim on the National team she was a medal winner in track as well. She was one of the original Canadian Paralympic athletes and had great success throughout her career. When I met her, she had won gold in the 60-metre sprint, and a silver in the slalom at the '68 Games in Mexico, plus a gold in the pool for winning the 25-metre freestyle event. She agreed with Bob on what he thought my classification might be, along with having a good insight into the competition that I would face if I did make it to the nationals. Both on the track and in the pool.

Can't say I ever enjoyed training or competing in the pool though. This body was not made for a Speedo! And freezing ranked second in discomfort. If I could have raced in hot water, who knows how good I could have been. Not great, but I would have been warm. Still, I trained all winter, but I was looking forward to getting on the track just a little bit more.

Chapter 2:
Let the Games Begin

Between school, basketball and swimming practise, the winter months went by quickly, and by the spring of '72, we got word that the Toronto Thrush Thunderbolts had been granted inclusion into the NWBA and would be playing in the Lake Erie Conference.

During our first practice, the guys had talked about the Detroit Sparks, kings of the conference, and that any skills we possessed, were nowhere near to what the 4-time defending NWBA Champions would bring to the court. We would also have to contend with two other teams that first year, the Toledo Silver Streaks and the Cleveland Comets. But league games were not until mid October, and a lot would happen before then.

While training seemed to be going well, my grades were no trip to Hollywood. The first two semesters were a general course, one where we were required to take classes delving into all aspects of media: working the cameras, running the boards in the booth for television, preparing slide presentations, all kinds of media related stuff. One course required working a certain number of hours on the college FM radio station. That's all I wanted to do, and it seemed like more than a few students in my classes only wanted to work in the areas that interested them as well.

Eventually it morphed into me doing multiple shows for multiple students on multiple days for hours on end. Especially in the dead of night. My reward was the notes from the classes I missed. However, it didn't really make up for not being there. They don't coddle you in college like they do in some small high school in the middle of nowhere, and stuff I handed in was so-so and it showed in my C average.

And with the end of the semester coming up in June, I had to find a place to live before the next term began in the Fall, since I was only supposed to rent a room at the McKee's for the first year. Bill and I got along so well that his mom said I could stay longer, and while I told my parents I had a new place, I just got in the habit of staying overnight at the college once I did move out.

Phase Two of Seneca was built with a common area that was huge and filled with couches and beanbag chairs. From an early age I've had the ability to sleep anywhere at anytime and it served me well until the semester ended.

And by now the custodians and I were good friends. Seneca was so new when I first enrolled, there was no elevator in Phase One to take me to the second floor for classes, and it ended up being the custodians that carried me up and down those two flights in my first two semesters. Those stairs were another reason why I preferred to stay on the main floor, where the school's FM radio station was.

After the semester was finished, and I was off for the summer, I planned to go back to Buckhorn. Mom and Dad had already decided to move to the cottage full-time and find something to do up there once they realized neither Dave nor I were interested in taking over the grocery store. With my high school girlfriend having moved on to bigger and better things, it meant I spent most of my time driving back and forth to Hamilton from Buckhorn. On the weekends, I would stay at Billy's parent's place in Kilbride, Brian's parent's place in Downsview, or I would sleep in the car.

So, I swam in the pool every Saturday with Billy and we met Bob at the McMaster University track every Sunday once the good weather finally arrived. Following Bob's lead, we did lap after lap on the track every weekend, and soon the Guelph Provincials were upon us.

The two things I remember most about my first provincial competition, was not how I fared in my events, but how a renewed friendship burst forth that first night before the competition had even started. And I remember the ordeal that was called classification.

On the day of registration, Billy, Brian and I were set to leave in convoy to the University of Guelph when one of our vehicles experienced engine problems before we could leave. By the time we stuffed everything into two cars, and we were ready to roll, we realized we might be late. Sure enough, it was dark when we arrived, and registration was closed until morning.

A large lounge in the university residence took up most of the main floor but our rooms were on the second, and there was no elevator. While we weighed our options, it was apparent that there was a party going on in more than one of the rooms on the second floor, and before long someone yelled down wondering what the hell was going on in the parking lot. I yelled up our predicament, but we had been prepared to sleep in the lounge or in our cars until morning if we had to. Imagine my surprise when someone stuck their head out of a window and called out "Is that Chris Stoddart?" It is so.

While most high school sports were beyond my level of adaptability, Arthur High had a wrestling team, and I was always grappling with the guys on the mats for fun during their practices or after school. Like trying to catch a chicken in the barnyard, I crawled around and made them work until ultimately, they "wrung my neck". But I had fun and while I was still a good fifteen pounds shy of my weight class maximum, I wanted to give it a try for real.

Both the Principal at the time, Mr. Brown and our Science teacher/wrestling coach, Mr. Hostrawser were open-minded enough to allow me to try out for the wrestling team. If, and it was a big if, my parents said it would be all right. Mom figured I'd be dead within the hour and there was no reasoning with her, so Dad stepped in to offer a compromise. Why don't we call my doctor and ask him if I can join the high school wrestling team? If he says yes, I'm good to go. Good ploy Dad, who would have thought the doctor would be on my side and say go ahead? Told my parents to let me try anything. If I got hurt, or it stopped being fun I would give it up and move on to something else. Wise advice for the 60's.

So, I joined the team and wrestled for the last couple of years of high school and made a few bus trips to other schools to wrestle. Wish I could say I was great, or even half bad, but I got pinned more than a few times and often outpointed when I did manage to stay out of trouble.

Starting from my hands and knees, I was already down by points to begin each match and wrestling in the old 98 lb Class at 75-80 pounds did not help much either. I did manage to pin a couple of skinny Grade 9ers from other schools to have some bragging rights, but regardless of my success on the mat, I was on the wrestling team and one of the guys. I don't remember any of the athletes I wrestled with back then except one, and I was in utter disbelief when I realized that that's who had called out my name.

Gordie Hope was a blind wrestler who went to school at the W. Ross MacDonald School for the Blind in Brantford in the 'Sixties, and he was someone I used to wrestle against in high school. The Brantford team bussed up to Arthur once a year and we would return the favour and get a bus trip down to Brantford and a day off school. Since we both normally wrestled regular guys that had eyesight and legs that worked, our matches were quite unique. A blind guy vs a gimp. Alien vs the Predator.

And here he was at these provincial games and how he recognized my voice, and the odds that he was at the same first competition was quite the surprise. But in a matter of minutes, a few of his larger buddies, all with limited or no eyesight mind you, worked their way down to the main floor and pulled us up the stairs to our rooms.

Gordie and I did not get a lot of sleep that night though, since I could not get over the fact that he could pick out my voice after all the time that had gone by.

In order to have a level playing field, everyone had to go through classification; a physical examination to ascertain their level of function. Bob had explained the process to me, since he had already gone through it before, so I thought I was pretty much prepared.

Not so. Sitting in your underwear on a gurney in one of any number of little makeshift examining rooms, while doctors poked and prodded and moved your legs all around in the attempt to determine your level of function, was not pleasant by any stretch of the imagination. While the process is relatively simple if you're a paraplegic as a result of an accident of some sort, and your impairment level is readily apparent, it's not near as cut and dried if you were born with a disability or contracted, say polio, early in life. Different disabilities manifest themselves in different ways and even two individuals with the same disability will often have completely different levels of impairment.

But regardless of how you ended up disabled, it was a degrading process, though unintentional on a certain level. In those early years I sometimes had

a near uncontrollable u[rge]
judgement prevailed fo[r]

So how were athlete[s]
on a chair. How's your
How far can you lean f[orward]
can you lean and no[t]
the way down, rest y[our]
back up to a sitting
stomach muscles to
how far can you lea[n]
same goes for your
did you have in y[our]
while you did the

If you had to push y[our]
of your wheelchair, you had a low classification
little or no functioning abdominals. If you could lean down part way [and]
straighten back up, you were in one of the higher classes. Every muscle that
you had, regardless of how weak it was, and regardless of if it played a part
in your event or not, was worth a point in the classification system. Low
overall points… one of the lower classes. Lots of points… upper classes. That's
an over-simplification of the process of course, but you get the general idea.

In the year that I first competed, the classification system had changed
from an A - B - C designation to a 1 - 2 - 3 system, Class 3 being the least
disabled of all the classes. Class 1 athletes were broken down even further.

If the athlete's disability also affected the upper torso and there was
reduced strength in the arms and hands, Class 1 was broken down into
1A - 1B - 1C, with 1A being the most disabled.

Over the course of my career, the classification system changed on more
than one occasion, and more classes added, as the emphasis turned towards
"useable muscles" in the act of doing the event, instead of the points system.

For the moment I was officially a Class 2 athlete. Billy was a Class 1 and
Bob remained a Class 3. The next level of classification would be waiting
for me in Calgary if I made the Ontario team. There the National team
doctors would have the final say before the competitions would begin.

and an eye-opener at the same time.
...en in a wheelchair, my legs had atrophied
... on crutches, I might have been in a higher
...ength I had in my legs had been drained away

...sure history could pinpoint the exact time that two indi-
...elchairs raced each other, the very act was inevitable. Man
...mpeting against one another since recorded time whether it be
... against one another, racing in chariots pulled by horses, or travel-
...undreds of miles an hour in mechanical contraptions of all sorts.

Who hasn't gone to the hospital at some point in their lives, either as a patient or a visitor, and hopped into a vacant wheelchair for a mad sprint down the corridor? I would imagine the veterans at Stoke Mandeville were racing each other the first chance they got.

To say the first wheelchairs we raced in, were racing chairs, would be comparable to saying the enthusiasts who raced their Chevys straight off the showroom floor were competing in race cars. We should have been so lucky. Our racing chairs were more like glorified shopping carts. What *was* similar, was the desire to get more speed out of what we had.

When wheelchair sports began, Stoke Mandeville rules specifically stated that the wheelchair must have four wheels and be built by a recognized wheelchair manufacturing company. Modifications were not permitted, but like the hotrodders of old, we soon learned how to tweak our machines to make them go faster, but I was pretty much racing "stock" in Guelph.

The Thunderbolts had quickly found me a smaller chair to play basketball in, and right away they had begun to cut it down. Most wheelchairs came with handles so you could be pushed around, and these were the first things that were cut off. As well, a high back on a chair made it difficult to reach around for a basketball that was thrown behind you, and that was the next part due for modification. The chair-back was cut down as far as it could while allowing the athlete to still maintain their personal level of balance. Although in some track competitions, removing the handles was considered a modification and could get your ride deemed illegal.

Chapter 2: Let the Games Begin

A lot of chairs came with removeable sides that were there to protect clothes from getting dirty or becoming stuck in the spokes. These were thrown away and the fittings were ground down smooth so that you didn't smash your thumb on them while pushing the chair.

It was hard to find a solid frame wheelchair because the vast majority were made to fold, to make transporting the chair in a vehicle easier. Problem with the folding wheelchair was that it rattled like a shopping cart, so one of the first "tricks" we used, was to tape the chair open, to help prevent it from flexing. It helped to a degree, but we still had a long way to go.

This chair was the first of many that I would use in competition. One chair for three functions. My everyday ride became a basketball chair once a front rollbar was attached, and then it transformed into a racing chair once you swapped out the front casters for 5" front wheels.

In the early years, you taped your fingers, wore gloves or wheeled barehanded. And while athletes from around the world began modifying their chairs, everyone had to be mindful of Stoke rules. Over the years as we continued to modify our chairs to go faster, and components were invented to help in that goal, many governing bodies around the world discouraged the advancements we wanted to make in chair design.

The competitions in Guelph were of course run with a great intent to do the best job possible, but back then, with lots of young volunteers with no experience, and a string stretched across the finish line, you can appreciate it was not at the level it is now. Each athlete was assigned someone with a stopwatch to record our times, but these times were subject to debate for the first couple of years. Be that as it may, Bob, Billy and myself won our 100 - 400 - and 1500 metre races, as did Hilda.

There were not a lot of athletes that first year in any of my events, but to my surprise I still won the discus - shot put and javelin competitions, as did Brian and Billy. Bob, by virtue of his standing in track, didn't have to worry about getting picked, so he got to relax.

While there were more swimmers to compete against in the pool, our results were the same and I managed to touch the wall first in all my events, as did Hilda and Billy.

In the end I had 10 shiny red FIRST PLACE ribbons when it was all said and done. I had never won a single ribbon in my whole life, including my high school days, before that day.

At the Closing Ceremonies, they announced the athletes that were going to represent Ontario at the 4th National Wheelchair Games in Calgary, scheduled for mid-June, and I was one of them! It was a lot to take in. We partied hard that night.

The next day there was a nice article in the Hamilton Spectator about the games, accompanied with a photo of a group of us posing with a basketball. First time I ever made the papers for winning a sporting event. This was all uncharted territory and still hard to believe.

Now that I was going to Calgary in a couple of weeks, I realized that I didn't have the money to pay my share of the registration fee that was required of each athlete going to the games. As Brian had said, money was scarce. While the provincial sports association was supplying some sponsorship, it was up to each athlete to come up with $90.00. It was money I didn't have, and I didn't want to ask my parents for it. I contemplated hitchhiking to Calgary but with all my gear, and even though I had already hiked out to Vancouver in my chair when I was younger, it didn't seem very practical that time around.

I mentioned my predicament to Coach Corrie and right away she called the mayor of the closest town to Buckhorn: Peterborough. After speaking to Douglas Gavin, the Mayor of Peterborough at the time, he arranged for me to meet that year's Rotarian-of-the-Year, Ed Meyer of the Peterborough Rotary Club. Just like that I had my first sponsor, and the only hurdle left was to bring back some hardware to show them the money was well spent.

The plane ride to Calgary was quite the experience. When I was younger, I had travelled to Sutton, a town in southern England to visit my mom's parents, but this was quite different. Loading that many disabled people onto an airplane was no easy feat and it took awhile before we had everything stored away and everyone carried on board that needed help. One thing I remember about flying as a team was how much we relied on all the coaches and support staff to get it done. Otherwise, it just would not have happened.

As most disabled people know, trying to find an accessible washroom, even nowadays, usually presents the biggest obstacle, regardless of where

Chapter 2: Let the Games Begin

you are travelling. Restaurants, arenas, you name it, especially in the '70s, were largely inaccessible, so finding one you could get your wheelchair into was a hit or miss thing. On a plane even more so. How our coaches picked up a 200-lb athlete, carried them down the aisle and squished them into what passed for a washroom doorway, and got them back out again, was beyond me. Luckily in my case, I just raced down the aisle on my hands and knees.

Once we landed in Calgary, the bus eventually pulled into the campus of the University of Calgary and my first big competition experience would begin.

After we unpacked, everyone headed for the hospitality tent to get reacquainted with friends. I soon realized that the "beer tent" was pretty much party central. If you were looking for something or someone, chances are success would be found in the beer tent. This was true even when we competed worldwide.

Being in the beer tent made me come to realize that, while everyone was super competitive and the good-natured trash talk between the provinces was constantly going on, the driving force of not only the athletes, but everyone involved, was the message they were trying to convey. A message that went way beyond the constrictions of our sport.

Sports was the venue we were using to show the world our worth. If we can do this, we can hold down jobs. Our disability does not make us incapable of leading regular productive lives. While I was never shy about putting my own two cents worth in on my own behalf growing up, this was different. This was not about me; we were showing the world the possibilities that were within us. Coming back from these games, whenever I was asked to talk about wheelchair sports or put on a demonstration, I was honoured to oblige.

First thing Bob and Billy did was seek out New Brunswick's Frank Henderson and over a couple of beers, they started filling his head about the new guy that they brought along who was going to blow him off the track. I bet Frank was thinking "Yah good luck with that".

Of course, before the competitions could begin, all the rookies had to go through classification again and after the examination by the National team doctors, we would be officially classified. Once through the ordeal again, I got an official ID card with my picture and my Class 2 designation printed on it.

If I ever harboured a crazy idea that I'd be coming home with a field medal, it was snuffed out quickly by this huge friendly guy that came over to introduce himself before the field events had begun. His name was Gene Reimer from B.C., already a multi-medal winner in numerous field events as a member of Canada's National team.

He didn't come over to tell me how good he was though, he just wanted to say welcome to the games and good luck. I would have needed more than luck that day. I think half of the field in my class could have tossed me farther than I could heave the shot! Long story short: no field event medals for me at the nationals. Ever.

Over in the pool, in my spiffy new red Team Ontario speedo, I checked out the competition. Toughest guy to beat would be Gunther Schuster of B.C. Pretty much a shark Hilda had told me. Gunther had been swimming for Canada since the beginning and would be a formidable challenge.

That year was not that different. He had one hiccup, when he had to settle for a silver in the 50-metre backstroke. I beat him to the wall, but I had to suck in pool water and barf at the end to get it done. He blew by me in all our other races though.

My first gold medal at the nationals and it was in the pool. Didn't see that coming! Still, Coach Corrie was going to be one happy camper once I got home. But as a swimming threat, the verdict was still out. I would need a lot of work to overcome Mr. Schuster or anyone else for that matter, on a regular basis.

As for the track, well apparently Frank wasn't softened up nearly enough because although I won 3 silvers, I was not able to really challenge him. While I did hold off veteran racer, Rene Massé from Quebec, Frank was untouchable.

He lowered his own Canadian 100 metre record down to 21.1 seconds while I settled for silver in 24.2. He slashed 20 seconds off the Canadian 400 metre record previously held by Orin Nordal of Manitoba, and his third gold netted him another national record by winning the 1500 metre in a time of 7:20.0, 9 seconds better than the record that was held by Duncan Wilson of B.C. I came in at 7:32.0. There was still a lot of work to be done.

Chapter 2: Let the Games Begin

While disappointed that I got "smoked", the best part about the experience was how nice a guy Frank was. No big ego either, no rubbing it in, not to me anyway, but I bet he got more than a couple of beers, compliments of the guys once our events were done. From then on, until he retired, we had a friendly rivalry, and we were destined to have an adventure of our own before the year was over.

I still had one more chance for a gold, as a member of the 240-metre relay team. Just like in able-bodied competitions, the relay is a hotly contested affair. In those early years, the relay was a 4 x 60 metre back-and-forth sprint that was contested on the track's front straightaway.

In this event, each team had 4 wheelies; at least 1 from each of the 3 classes, and a 4th from any Class of the team's choosing. The Ontario team was a strong one and although Frank was lightning fast, the New Brunswick team was not the reigning champions. The toughest challenge would come from British Columbia, anchored by Class 3 Pete Colistro, and included Gene Reimer as well. Even though Gene made his mark in field events, his success in the pentathlon meant he was plenty quick in the sprint as well.

The relay was set up with each team assigned 2 side-by-side lanes, 2 athletes at each end of the 60-metre straightaway. When the gun went off, your leadoff man raced 60 metres up the track, and tagged his teammate between the shoulder and the elbow within the exchange area. That athlete wheeled back to the finish where he tagged the team's third racer, and that athlete raced back up the track to tag the anchor man, who raced back to the finish line.

I led off, followed by Billy, and Thunderbolt teammate Mike O'Brien. Bob wheeled the anchor. We were fast enough to upset the BC squad and Ontario had its first national gold medal in the relay since the National Games had begun.

I entered 12 events all told in Calgary, including playing on the provincial basketball and volleyball teams, but there was one event contested in Calgary that was not offered in Ontario. It was called the slalom and it was a timed obstacle course that you raced through. It was intended to highlight the dexterity, manoeuverability and speed of the wheelchair athlete.

There were pylons to go though, both forward and backwards. A ramp led to a platform where you had to do a 360 degree turn on top. You were required to jump up a curb and bump down the other side. There was usually a short straightaway that took you to the finish line.

Each athlete went through the course, one at a time, the order based on the number you drew out of a hat. If you touched a pylon, there was a time penalty. If you missed something entirely, you ended up disqualified. It was a unique event in that there were no heats, fastest time wins, and you got one crack at it. Watching it I thought this event was right up my alley, being small and all. Next year perhaps.

As I soon came to realize, time goes by quickly and suddenly the games were over and we were all sitting at a table at the Closing Ceremonies and Awards Banquet. To my amazement, my showing was enough to win the Male Rookie-of-the-Year Award.

I donated the new wheelchair that I received for winning, back to the Calgary charity that had put it up as the prize. It was too big for me, and I knew it would be much more useful for someone else. Besides, this chair was fine. It was time to tinker. I had spotted some things on other chairs and that gave me something to think about going forward. Time would tell if my ideas would help.

Then the big news came. I made the Paralympic team going to West Germany for the 21st Stoke Mandeville Games in August. I was set to become a Paralympian. I couldn't believe it! To say I dreamed of this moment would be a boldfaced lie. Growing up disabled, I never once dreamed that I'd be an athlete, let alone one that was destined to represent their country.

Came back home from Calgary basking in the glory of it all and still marvelling at the fact that I was a member of the Canadian Paralympic Team. My parents were thrilled, I got a blurb in my hometown paper, the Arthur Enterprise, and my new girlfriend in Buckhorn had something to brag about. Things were good.

Though I did realize that an article about you in a newspaper is not *always* a good thing, even with the best intentions. Just back from Calgary, an un-named newspaper wrote a glowing account of my success out west. The first paragraph said, in part: "Chris Stoddart of Buckhorn, College graduate, International Paralympic competitor… and life-long cripple".

Chapter 2: Let the Games Begin

Now while my first reaction was to laugh out loud, my Dad threw what I used to call a *hairy fit*. It took a while for Mom to talk him out of driving down into the city and shoving the newspaper. Well, you get the idea.

When the guys read the article, they laughed as well and for a while, if any of us got too detailed while explaining a basketball victory or something "great" that we did, someone would chime in with… " and life-long cripple". That never failed to get a reaction!

I had no idea that I would be in this position going into Calgary and now that I was slated to go to Germany in August, I had to come to terms with what it really meant. While I was currently off for the summer, school was slated to start back up while I was in Germany. Not only would I be out of the country for the games, but I intended to go on the 3-week bus tour of Europe that some of the athletes were going on after the competitions concluded. If I missed the beginning of the semester, I would have to wait a whole year to get back in. What to do?

It was a no-brainer really! Who turns down a chance to represent their country on their sports biggest stage? I was so excited to race. And really, I had no idea if I would ever get another chance. For all I knew this trip might be my only opportunity. So, I decided. School could wait, and it did.

When the Rotary Club of Peterborough found out I made the team going to Germany, they paid for my trip to the games and for the bus trip afterwards. As well, the neighbours that lived around my parents in the Buckhorn Hideaway passed the hat around and presented me with a nice card signed by everyone, and some spending money for when I was on the tour. In the blink of an eye, it seemed, we were all at Pearson Airport getting ready to fly to England and on to Germany.

The plane ride was long and uncomfortable, but we eventually made it to England and then on to Heidelberg. A bus took us to our accommodations and once we had unpacked our gear, we wheeled around and took it all in.

The Games had been scheduled to be held in Munich after the Summer Olympics, but the Olympic Village was scheduled for renovations once the Olympics were over, and when accommodations couldn't be found, the Paralympics were moved to the University of Heidelberg and its Institute for Physical Training.

Most fortunate for me was the fact that Bob and I were roommates. I learned a lot from him in those days we spent together. No doubt he helped mold me into the athlete I would become, especially on the mental side of things.

As I mentioned before, he was the undisputed fastest wheelie, by virtue of his record 19 second wheel in the 100 metres. The times for all the other classes in the 100 metres were in the low 20 seconds and were destined to stay that way for more than a few years. Bob blew a tendon in his arm during that race and had to fly home early, but he did what he had set out to do. And this time he was planning to be champion once more.

There in our room he began to tell me his strategy. Focus on the task at hand. Do not get distracted. And how did he stay focused?

Well as we were unpacking, he pulled out a large bottle of Southern Comfort and stuck it on the table. I knew the hospitality tent would be opening soon, but weren't we rushing things just a little bit? Not really. The bottle was to stay there until he won the 100 metres. Then he would crack it open, and we would all get a swig to celebrate.

Sounded good to me, except it was in plain view of anyone walking past our room and it wasn't long before one of our coaches strolled past and saw the bottle. It was obvious that the two of them had been to other competitions together because he came in our room and they started talking about the facilities and how good the accommodations were, compared to other places they had been.

But eventually the topic got around to the bottle and Bob explained that he brought it with him to celebrate winning the 100 metres. "Fair enough", says the coach, "But does it have to sit there in full view of everyone walking by?"

So, it was moved to the table between our beds, and it stayed there waiting, as a reminder. Focus. Always remember to focus.

One of the most important lessons I ever learned in all my years of competing and one that has never left me...has never diminished its impact...has in fact grown stronger over time...was the sense of unbelievable affection that countries in Europe have for Canadians.

This came to me at Opening Ceremonies, during the parade of athletes when suddenly, as the announcer called out "Canada", the stands erupted

Chapter 2: Let the Games Begin

and scared the life out of me. Thunderous applause rained down on us and I found myself getting emotional.

Having gone through the opening ceremonies in Calgary, I had an idea of what to expect. We would parade around the track and then sit in groups, this time in countries instead of provinces. A bunch of officials would make speeches and declare the games open. Cool, it was exciting, make no mistake. Representing my country half-way around the world was the greatest thing that had ever happened to me, so I was stoked.

But I was not prepared for the reaction that greeted the announcement of Canada's presence to the packed stands. Aside from the home country, no other country got the response that our team did. People were on their feet, cheering like we had already won something. As I was wheeling along, I started to shake, and I confess to having tears in my eyes.

I looked at Bob with questions on my face. He noticed my demeanor and laughed, but he was serious when he said it's because they don't forget. The people of Europe will never stop appreciating what we did for them during the War. We asked for nothing in return and acted like it was no big deal. No, they will love Canadians forever... and that's why it's so important to always act the proper way, before, during and after the games are over. We have a lot to live up to. Never make us look bad.

Suffice to say I came back from Europe with a much greater appreciation, and a broader understanding of what really went on back then and a little insight into what my dad must have gone through as a member of the 48th Highlanders fighting in Europe and Italy.

In time, being married to a woman whose father was a decorated tail-gunner that managed to cram his large frame into the belly of a Halifax bomber, and from working for the War Amputations of Canada for 27 years until my retirement in 2010, all that has given me a thorough knowledge and appreciation for all the sacrifices that our Armed Forces made for our freedom.

Race day finally arrived, and it was not what everyone was hoping for. The rain that started on day one had only gotten worse as the week went on. The hard-packed clay track turned into a sea of mud. The longer races were cancelled, and everyone set their sights on the 100 metre and the relays. Now it was time to watch another lesson unfold, thanks to Bob.

The rain outside found me taking my time getting onto the track. It was still pouring down, windy and cold. I was not looking forward to wheeling in these conditions. Over the years, being so light, the wind has affected my ability to go fast on more than one occasion and has cost me winning medals along the way. Coupled with all the mud, things were not going to be easy. Not at all.

As I got closer, I saw Bob under one of the trees, off by himself, smoking a cigarette. Obviously, he had been told to kick the habit by coaches since he first started racing, but his opinion was that the day he got beat he'd quit racing for good... otherwise.

Everyone else was down at the track, freaking out about the conditions and how the times were going to be slow etc. But, while wheelers from other countries were trying to get some speed up going through the mud during race day's practise time, Bob sat on a cushion under the tree, and smoked cigarettes. Relaxed.

When he saw me, he called me over, "Get out of the rain and get comfortable", he said. "Don't go on the track, it's a waste of time. All you're going to accomplish is to get all kinds of mud on your chair and inside the wheel bearings. Worse, if your hand slips on a muddy hand-rim and you pull a muscle, you're done. Relax. Sit and watch."

So, we sat there. It was a good idea really. Not like it is now; we didn't have a fancy hi-tech chair that we climbed into to race. Gumming up the chair from slogging through the mud meant it would probably have seized bearings eventually. Probably somewhere in Europe on the bus trip, with my luck.

While others were attempting to wheel through the mud, I noticed that a few athletes were watching us from the track. Bob just sat there smoking and watching them struggle. And looking at the guys who were looking at him. Not an "evil eye" kind of stare, he just gave off the impression that he was not worried in the slightest.

Sitting there, relatively warm and comfortable, I asked him why he made a point of sitting there smoking instead of going inside and relaxing. He said because when you are the man to beat, and you're sitting there

Chapter 2: Let the Games Begin

smoking, it gives the competition something to think about. How can he smoke and be that fast? And so, he smoked in front of them to put it in their heads that he could afford to sit there and smoke a pack a day if he felt like it.

They already knew he was the one to beat. He had wheeled a good two seconds faster in the 100 than anyone else in any class had gone. Two seconds is an eternity in the 100. And while everyone knew there was not going to be any records set on this track, nonetheless he gave the impression that he was not worried about the outcome in the slightest.

He smiled a lot while we were under that tree. In fact, he told me he was happy it was miserable. Use the bad weather to your advantage. Another lesson learned. The conditions were bad, but they were bad for everyone. The more you stressed on it, the more impact it would have on your performance. He couldn't understand why more athletes didn't take that into consideration. If it's raining, wear rain gear. If it's cold, race in warmer clothes. It isn't always going to be clear sunny skies. And regardless of the circumstances, act like it's no problem. Yes, I learned a lot from Bob on that trip.

Eventually I found myself in Lane 4, on the starting line for my qualifying heat in the 100 metres, in the biggest competition in the world. My heart was moving at a good clip, even before the gun went off.

Boom... and away I went. I tried to remember what Bob said. Look nowhere but straight ahead. Focus. Be sure to push past the finish line.

I did all that and won by about 8 chair lengths. Good for the semi-finals. Frank pounded his way down the track and won his heat by a large margin as well. So far so good.

But... not so fast. After all the heats for all the classes of both men and women were completed, the track was a deep sea of mud, so instead of semi-finals, the top 8 times would go directly to the final. Frank and I were 9th and 10th.

And Bob? He did just exactly what he said he would do. Set the fastest qualifying time and then destroyed the field in the final on the way to his gold medal. All according to plan. That night we celebrated his still being the quickest man alive in a chair. But I could never drink Southern Comfort again.

While Frank and Bob, with help from Gene Reimer and Nova Scotia's Walter Dann, went home with a silver from their efforts in the relay, I left with a wealth of new knowledge and a feeling about myself that had never reached those heights before. I was a real Paralympian.

Bob wasn't the only track athlete to come home with a medal though. Edmonton's Doug Bovee won gold in the Class 1A slalom and a silver in the 60-metre sprint.

On the women's side, Hilda took silver in the Class 3 slalom and another silver in the 60-metre sprint plus a bronze in the pentathlon. Hilda's best friend, Sharon Long, won bronze in the Class 1B slalom.

In the pool, Canada took home a couple of medals. Richard Wasnock of BC won the gold in the 75-metre medley and Veronica Demerakas took home bronze in her 25-metre backstroke event.

My results in the pool produced finishes in the 7th and 8th place range, and I was not encouraged by those mediocre results. Going home ranked 10th in the world in the 100 was much more exciting. I was proud of myself, but I had work to do once I got back home. I won my heat, and I was happy about that, but it only made me determined to get faster.

With the Paralympics completed, part of the team prepared for the trip back to Canada while those of us who were staying to go on the bus tour of Europe, made ready. The itinerary had us heading to Munich, Innsbruck, Zurich, Interlaken, Geneva, Dijon and finally on to Paris.

And no doubt, it was on this trip that I forged my reputation for doing crazy things. But what can I say, I was twenty-one and loose on another continent. It was time to have some fun, Stoddart Style.

It's a no brainer that pictures, and lots of them, are required for having a great trip. Not only for yourself to reminisce over, but to show your friends and family the people and places you encountered during your adventures. Since we didn't have cell phones with built-in cameras, and all the other fancy electronic gadgets we have now, we were only armed with a Polaroid or a trusty 35mm camera.

A nice opportunity presented itself while we were going through the mountains in Germany, I believe. The scenery was breathtaking as we worked our way up and down the various mountain roads. Eventually we came to a kind of rest stop with a great view of a deep canyon with an old, old castle on the far side. Just beautiful. Gorge deeper than I thought possible. Millions of tons of rock carved over the millennia by the river now hundreds of feet below.

There was a rock barrier that you could stand along to take pictures, but it was impossible to see to the bottom of the gorge while sitting in a wheelchair. The barrier was to naturally prevent people from getting too close to the edge and toppling off. Still, I wanted a better picture if I could get one, and a tree off to the side there seemed sturdy enough and its branches stretched out over the abyss. What were the chances it would snap under my puny weight if I shinnied up and out a little bit to take a few pictures?

With a little help with distraction from an unnamed accomplice, I grabbed a few cameras, hung them over my neck, and with a boost by someone... don't ask who... I was up the tree, had snapped a few pictures and was back before the coaches knew what I was up to.

Well almost all of them. So, I took heat for, you know, going crazy, potentially dropping to my doom for a couple of pictures, scaring the crap out of everyone. I promised I'd never do such a dumb thing again. And I never hung from a tree over a gorge for the whole rest of the trip. A promise is a promise. And by the way, none of my pictures turned out, so if anyone out there has one, consider yourself lucky!

Not to say the fun was over though. One day we found ourselves in Zurich for a day or so. Plenty of time to go sight-seeing, so a small group of us headed out to look around. The city is so old. It reeks of time. Every weather-beaten piece of rock seemed to be full of stories of times past.

As we wheeled/walked along one of the streets, we came across this old bridge that spanned the river that flowed about 20 feet below. The sides were made of rock and concrete and formed identical half circles that rose another good 20 or 30 feet on either side.

Looked amazing. Time for a picture. But while looking at it, I concluded that the arc of the sides of the bridge were not all that steep. As well, they were about two feet wide and smooth on top. If one were careful, one could work their way up the side to the top, take some great pictures, and then work their way down to the other side of the bridge.

'Course I needed help to pull it off. Someone would have to sit in my chair and wheel across the bridge so that it was there when I descended, and no-one saw an empty chair if they looked around. No problem. Always someone there to give me a hand.

A few of us hung back a bit and in a blink of an eye, the switch was made, and I was on the ledge and making steady progress. It was kind of windy as I climbed higher, so I had to concentrate on going slow and methodical. Pretty much dark by the time I reached the top, and as it turned out, my pictures showed nothing distinguishable when I had them developed back home. Different shades of murky blackness. I sense a pattern here!

Going down proved to be a lot more of a challenge though. The concrete was smooth all right, but somehow looking downward, the arc looked to be a lot steeper than it did looking up. A couple of times, I slid forward just enough to make my heart jump. I realized I'd have to slow down and not let any momentum build up, or I was liable to slide off onto the road, or maybe worse, drop an extra 20 into the river. But I made it down. Another successful stunt pulled off, but not everyone was impressed.

Things were pretty much uneventful after that. In fact, I was thinking that to myself one day, as we were all enjoying a boat ride in a type of sightseeing boat during one of our stops along the way. Like a massive houseboat, it had room to walk all around the outside of the centre structure that housed the kitchen, the main dining room, and the bridge. You could also climb up the stairs to the roof for a more panoramic view. Breathtaking.

It had three metal railings that went completely around the boat, and I was quite relaxed and enjoying the view, until someone ventured that it might be possible to hang from the top railing of the cabin, and hand-walk their way around the whole boat without falling into the river. Anyone interested? Ah well, I was confident that this one would be a piece of cake.

Turns out, it was one of my easiest stunts. Never fell in the river, didn't even get winded. Never came close to letting go, even when one of our team officials suddenly pulled back the curtain to check out the view as he had lunch, only to see me smiling at him as I made my way past the dining room windows. They all laughed. That's just Stoddart, doing something crazy.

Chapter 2: Let the Games Begin

I wheeled straight for most of the rest of the trip. I refrained from any stunts but ultimately Fate would lead me, and my teammate Frank, on the biggest adventure of all. And we just wanted to see the Eiffel Tower.

We were in Paris, on the last leg of our trip, and I had promised my girlfriend before I left Canada, that I'd do something "romantic" for her while I was there. I had decided that it would be cool to draw a heart with our initials on the Tower as a sign of our never-ending love (or until the end of the summer as Fate would have it) and place a Canadian coin somewhere in one of the cracks. I'd be in jail nowadays for defacing a national treasure, but no-one cared almost fifty years ago.

Frank and I headed out from our hotel in our chairs in the early afternoon, just as the hotel manager came on for the day. He gave us general directions to the Tower but stressed it was a long way. Bah, we are strong athletes, and so off we went.

We were prepared to wheel whatever the distance was, but how hard could it be to find what we were looking for? It was the Eiffel Tower for heaven's sake. Like standing in downtown Toronto and trying to find the CN Tower. Or so we thought.

We wheeled for a few hours in the direction we thought we were supposed to be headed. By late afternoon we began to casually ask people directions to the Tower. "Looking for the Eiffel Tower". "Can you point us in the direction of the Eiffel Tower?" "Have you heard of the Eiffel Tower?" People looked at us like we were high on something. Eventually we came to the Seine River, crossed over and started following it, still asking about a tower that seemingly no-one had ever heard of, and we hadn't even glimpsed in our travels.

By now a good three, going on four hours had passed since we left the hotel and we seemed to be no closer to our goal, but we had decided that we were not stopping until we found the Tower. If we had to take a cab back to the hotel, fine, but we were not giving up.

Eventually, lo and behold, we met a guy that spoke English. For the love of everything holy, where is the Eiffel Tower?!! "Oh, you mean La Tour Eiffel?" "It's about 10 miles that way", as he pointed in another direction. So that's it? La Tour Eiffel? None of the people we asked could figure out where we wanted to go? No... he said, we were obviously tourists of the common type.

Call our famous landmark by its proper name and pronunciation or do without. Well, thank you kindly. And where is our hotel? Back the other way.

By now we were beginning to run out of daylight, but we were still determined to find the Tower. And we figured we knew a shorter way back to the hotel.

It was virtually dark when we finally wheeled up to the structure. True to my word I etched our initials in the base of the Tower and squeezed a Canadian nickel into one of the cracks in the foundation. Mission accomplished. No time to marvel at the structure though. Time to get back. The hard part was about to begin.

We had a long way to go and wandering the streets of Paris in the dark was not a safe thing to do, especially near the river and the docks. But by now we thought we knew the shortest route back to the hotel (which we didn't), and we wheeled along at a good pace. The one time we saw figures moving towards us out of the dark, as we were wheeling along the Seine, we picked up our pace even more and we weren't followed for long.

Wheeled for hours but we kept on going, and with the sun coming up, we realized we had found the street that the hotel was on, and eventually it came into view.

Bone tired and caked in dirt we wheeled into the lobby. The same gentleman that saw us off, was still manning the desk and was beside himself when he realized we were just getting back. It's dangerous at night he said. We believe you.

And it seemed our roommates had covered for us because as we were explaining our route, a couple of our coaches came out of the elevator. They did look at us funny but probably thought we had just gotten back from an early morning wheel. The streets of Paris back then were not the cleanest. Either way, off they went. The Manager came around with a map of Paris and he traced the route we described.

The map revealed we had wheeled through Paris like drunken sailors and were getting close to the Tower a couple of times before veering off in the wrong direction. That map is at home, framed and mounted with the rest of my sports memorabilia.

And other than sleeping in the overhead storage compartment on the way back across the Atlantic and causing a bit of a panic when the head

Chapter 2: Let the Games Begin

count was off, I was a good boy. I had lots to think about and a lot of training to do if I were to ever beat Frank or ultimately win a medal for Canada. We were all looking forward to the '73 Nationals in Vancouver, a stepping-stone in preparation for the next set of Paralympics.

But basketball would begin in a month or so and the anticipation of playing in the NWBA was high. We were about to make history, though at the time I'm not sure we genuinely appreciated the significance in terms of the growth of wheelchair basketball in the province that this step meant. I was just looking forward to seeing how good this team called the Detroit Sparks really were.

Coming back to Canada, I planned to stay at my parent's place in Buckhorn for the winter months while I decided what to do during my downtime from college. But it wasn't long before I got a job offer from Bell Canada in October.

At the time, my brother Dave was working for Bell Telephone and while I was away, they ran a nice article in their newspaper about him and his disabled brother who was competing for Canada in Germany. They knew I had to forgo school for a year, and they called and asked if I would like a job in Directory Assistance, at the Toronto Bell Building at Yonge and Eglinton in the meantime.

I would be working in the Rate & Route Department, a job which required an operator to answer questions like how much a call would cost from point A to point B, among a host of other tasks. There were all kinds of directories to go through to come up with the answers.

I would be the only guy in a group of maybe 30 women of all ages including my bosses. Did I have a problem with any of it? Hell no. All the ladies to myself? Looking forward to it. I was unattached again, having learned my lesson. Don't come home empty-handed from a competition after your girlfriend has talked you up to all her friends. Eiffel Tower? Big deal.

But taking the job meant having to find a place to live since I couldn't very well drive back and forth from beyond Peterborough everyday and expect to hold down a full-time job. But again, through Disability Assistance, an apartment was found for me in the newly finished St. James Town complex. It was a great place and a couple of Thunderbolt teammates had apartments in the complex as well. And with our first season in the NWBA about to begin, living in Toronto made it a lot easier to get to practice and train for the next set of games.

I also bought my first car to get back and forth to work. A new metallic brown '72 Pontiac Ventura hatchback with a big-block 350 engine. That car went like the wind, and I kick myself for selling it, every time I think about her.

Those of us who had competed in the summer were in good shape, and ready to begin practising when the '72/'73 ball season rolled around. Being on the first wheelchair basketball team from Ontario and only the second in all of Canada to play in the NWBA, we were all excited to start and make a good showing, regardless of how good the competition was.

A great thing about the Calgary Nationals was the experience gained from being a member of the provincial basketball team and watching the fierce rivalries that had already been formed between the provinces. Ontario had never won a basketball medal at the nationals. British Columbia had won 9 out of the first 10 National Championships, thanks in no small part to a team that was made up of most of the players from the NWBA Vancouver Cable Cars. They were a strong team and almost always made it a dogfight among the other Western provinces to see who would meet them in the final. Playing for a basketball medal became part of my focus looking forward to the Vancouver Nationals to be held the following summer.

But back to the task at hand. The question now was, how badly would we lose to the teams in our conference going into our first season? Brian had told me repeatedly that we were going to be way over our heads in the beginning, but after watching the talent in Calgary, I wondered how much better could the Detroit Sparks be?

Our Thunderbolt uniforms were dark blue, with THUNDERBOLTS lettered in an arc across the front. Underneath was a round crest, featuring the Thrush Muffler woodpecker logo, our original team sponsor. Our numbers were on the back.

The first game in the history of the team was played against the Detroit Sparks on November 14th, 1972, at the Stevenson High School in Livonia Michigan.

The site of this game was fitting, I think, since we got schooled in the game of wheelchair basketball, as they were way better than I could have

Chapter 2: Let the Games Begin

imagined. In ball control, ball movement, heck pretty much in every aspect of the game, they showed us how it was supposed to be played. And of course, they were all fast on the court. We lost 102-27.

They went around us and scored, blew by us and scored, passed back and forth and scored, or shot over us and scored. But with a big lead, the law of averages will tip to your side eventually, and during a couple of their momentary lapses, I managed to get away for a couple of fast-break buckets. My third basket resulted in legendary Sparks' coach Bud Rumple staring down his teammate who was supposed to be covering me. "If you can't stop the *Roadrunner*, I'll find someone who can". Enough said. I acquired a shadow, and I was not afforded another opportunity that day. But I had a new nickname. Not bad either, the bird and I were almost the same size. I felt it was an improvement over *Spider*.

We lost all 4 games against Toledo but upset Cleveland 42-35 for our first NWBA win when we travelled to Ohio for the Saturday night game. Though we lost on the Sunday game, we were a happy group when we headed back to Canada. Cleveland won the first game up here in Canada but forfeit the second to get a head start back home when a snowstorm was forecast for the Sunday.

We finished with a 2-10 record but steadily improved as the years past. The Thunderbolts played in the NWBA until our last season of '78/'79. We never did beat the Sparks, but we got much better, and a lot of great ball players got their start as members of the 'Bolts.

Chapter 3:
One Step Forward –
One Step Back

With winter almost gone, I was itching to getting outside on a track. So as soon as it was free of snow, I met Bob and Billy every Sunday afternoon back at the McMaster track and we would begin our routine of as many laps as we could. Just varied our speed depending on the distance we were trying to replicate. And I still did laps in the YWCA pool.

The Provincials Wheelchair Games came around in May and were held at the University of Waterloo in Kitchener. With no new athletes in our class to go against, the three of us were once again picked for the Vancouver Nationals, scheduled to run from mid-May to the beginning of June. We would be racing on the track at the University of British Columbia. With some hard work in the meantime, I hoped it would help me give Frank a wheel for his money.

In life, sometimes wonderful things happen to you out of the blue and it changes everything about who you are and the capabilities that are hidden within you. This happened to me a couple of weeks before we were to leave for Vancouver, and it began a pattern that followed me throughout my whole career. Before I would leave for a national competition, something major would happen in my life, both good and bad. This time it was very good.

I was taking a break to drink some water when I was approached by a man who asked me what I was doing. Training for the upcoming nationals I explained, and I gave him a short version of the whole wheelchair sports experience. He asked me what kind of training I did, and I said laps, lots of laps.

As it turned out his name was Graham Ward, and he was an associate professor at McMaster University and one of the coaches of the Hamilton Olympic track team that trained on this very same track. How would I like a real track coach? He ventured that he could make me a lot faster if all I did was laps. That was enough for me. At that moment, I had just become the first wheelchair racer in Canada at least, to have his own coach and be trained like an able-bodied athlete. With Billy and Bob on board, we were looking forward to Graham's help.

Eventually, after more than a decade, Graham had helped numerous Canadian racers achieve their ultimate goals. By 1982 he was the Track & Field Co-Ordinator for our National Team, and in 1984 he would be the Canadian National Team coach and the Sports Director at the famous Variety Village facility in Scarborough. There is no way I would have achieved the success I did without everything he did for me. Over the years, many track athletes benefitted from his training as well. But in the beginning, our little group reaped the benefits of his forward thinking.

The Nationals in Vancouver were held as part of the BC Festival of Sports that ran all through the summer of '73, and you would have thought that I was going to find myself closer to Mr. Henderson than I was the year before. However, Vancouver did not turn out the way I had envisioned. Even with Graham beside me, it unravelled before my eyes.

Sophomore jinx, bad luck, me being a total screw-up, take your pick. I didn't show the Selection Committee much, and while Billy would eventually venture down to South American for the Pan Am Games and come home with a silver medal, the only place I travelled that year was back home.

Got too excited in the 100 and false started. Tried too hard on the re-start and as a result of trying to catch up to Frank, who had already built an insurmountable lead, I veered out of my lane, impeded another racer and was disqualified. One down.

I won a silver in the 400, but I was 8 seconds behind, and in the 1500 I was unable to hold off Rene Massé in the final stretch and had to settle for a bronze. On the last day of racing, Bob, Billy, myself and veteran Ron Thompson took home a bronze in the 240-metre relay.

Though the slalom was still not offered at the provincial level, I really liked the event when I was in Calgary the year before, and I made sure I was signed up to compete this time around. Over the years, the slalom would become one of my most successful events.

In the early years, the course was unique to each competition, provincially and nationally. More than a few of Canada's fast track guys wheeled the slalom as well. Some did great, others not so much, but once more distances were added to the race schedule, only the athletes who found themselves on the slalom podium regularly continued entering this event.

Being small, I did have an advantage since the gates were a regulation distance apart, so the wider your chair was, the less room you had for error, and the most important thing was to wheel a penalty-free run. If your chair touched anything it shouldn't, it was a 3-second penalty. You can cover a lot of distance in 3 seconds. Touching pylons usually spelt disaster unless others did the same. Wheeling through clean when it was your turn, was a big advantage to have and one that the other competitors to follow would have on their minds.

There were a lot of competitors in this event at these nationals, but I managed to win the silver medal. I was hooked. This was as much fun as racing on a track.

Over in the pool, I did come away with a gold medal, winning the 50-metre backstroke, and a silver in the 50-metre freestyle, and I *was* quicker than the year before, but I still could not get enthused about swimming. But if it continued to help get me a berth on the national team, I was still willing to continue.

The first time I was asked if I would like some "help", was during these Vancouver Nationals. It was suggested to me that I needed to put on weight and some muscle if I was going to ever beat Frank or anyone else.

You might be surprised that the use of performance enhancing drugs in wheelchair sports is not as cut and dried a subject as you might think. The main fact being a drug policy wasn't put in place in Canada at least, until the early '80s, more than a decade after the formation of disabled sports.

Chapter 3: One Step Forward – One Step Back

There are numerous reasons for that, the first being than the involvement in sports for the disabled, was aimed at rehabilitation in the beginning. How well you did, how fast you wheeled your hospital chair, or how well you shot a basketball, was irrelevant in the big scale of things. It was all aimed at getting the individual as healthy as possible. Physically, by engaging in activity, and mentally; since playing with other individuals in the "same boat" as you helped keep the spirits up to continue to get better. But if you were competitive enough and wanted to win bad enough, it was there for the taking. You could take what you wanted if you wanted to.

Coming from a non-competitive sports background, I didn't know anything about steroids, and I just didn't believe that taking chemicals would make me as big as the other guys.

My fear of needles and my inability to take pills unless I crushed them into a fine powder before eating them, made me pass on that approach as well. And even though I was gung-ho to beat Frank, I didn't care that much about coming out on top if I had to go through that kind of stuff to do it. I had enough pills and needles growing up to last a lifetime. Doing it on purpose did not appeal to me in the slightest.

Over time, I realized that the idea of an even playing field was more an allusion regardless of how accurate the classifications were, or whether you were *clean* or not, when I mentioned the exchange to Graham when we got back home to Ontario.

Relieved that I had turned down the offer, he had a few words of advice for me going forward. He explained that there were big athletes and small athletes, nothing could change that fact, and that's why he encouraged me to concentrate on getting *myself* better, getting *myself* faster. There was nothing I could do if I got beat by a bigger athlete, who's fitness level was the same as mine. He had a bigger engine and unless my "power-to-weight" ratio was such that it could overcome the extra strength and energy that the bigger athlete had at his disposal, victories would be difficult to achieve. Graham felt my power-to-weight ratio and better technique were my two best options going forward. I needed to concentrate on getting myself better. If my best meant I got a medal, good for me. It was sage advice.

Not to mention, competing around the world gave you an up-close view of the life that other disabled individuals lived, in places that had none of the advantages we had in Canada. No fancy racing chair was one obvious difference. Often athletes from other countries used each other's chair to compete in. In later years, even when we had a regular chair, a racing machine and a basketball chair, many athletes around the world still had one chair for everything.

When you added poor nutrition, lack of training and facilities to train in, it was hard to see an even playing field. But against yourself? Make that your priority and you should do fine.

But as the years past, athletes got fitter and more competitive, and as equipment got better, those in the sport in Canada and throughout the world, started to press the point that we were legitimate athletes and the sport had evolved to the point that we needed to be recognized as such. No longer were we individuals that competed to show the world our off-track capabilities. We felt we had achieved that already. Now we wanted to be recognized for what we felt we had become. Real athletes. Not wheelchair athletes, not blind or amputee athletes, but athletes who trained like their able-bodied counterparts. Like cyclists, who had progressed from racing on ordinary bikes to racing machines worth thousands of dollars, our chairs had evolved over time from the clunky hospital chairs into custom made racers. And the transformation had just begun.

However, when we began to ask for government funding and began the process of getting recognition of our sport as being legitimate, it brought up the question of drug testing. If we were to be recognized and funded as athletes in our own right, we needed to be under the same rules as all able-bodied athletes. And that meant being clean.

Unfortunately, there were some who were not able to follow the guidelines. Glory is one thing for an athlete to strive for, but the promise of cold hard cash and sponsorships were dangling carrots that over the years, became too much to resist for some.

For me, I trained for the rest of that summer and had forgotten the disappointment of Vancouver by the time October rolled around, and another ball season was at hand.

Chapter 4:
A Taste of Success

Soon as the weather permitted, I was on my way to Hamilton, Saturday in the pool, and Sunday afternoons at McMaster, where Graham put us through our paces.

After my poor showing in Vancouver left me off the '73 Pan Am Team, I vowed to make up for it at the '74 mid-August Winnipeg Nationals. And with Graham's training, I was going a lot faster than I ever had before. How fast? That remained to be seen. And more importantly I still had to do well enough at the provincials, slated for Belleville in June.

We had already begun to see the benefits of real training though, as lap after lap had been replaced with something called interval training.

This consisted of hard repeated runs of 100 to 1500 metres with 80% effort. We got enough rest in between to allow for another 80% effort. As we got fitter, the rest period decreased. By taxing our body anaerobically, we also benefitted by wheeling with better form and with a higher top speed.

Before the provincials, Gene Reimer and I were present at the press conference in Toronto that announced the awarding of the '76 Paralympics, formally to be known as the TorontOlympiad, to be held at Centennial Park in August of '76 in Etobicoke.

The Chairman of the Organizing Committee was Canada's Dr. Robert Jackson, an orthopedic surgeon at Toronto General Hospital and who had been the orthopedic consultant to the Canadian Olympic Team in Tokyo in 1964. I personally consider him to be Canada's equivalent of Sir Ludwig Guttmann for being the moving force behind the formation of the

Canadian Wheelchair Sports Association in 1967, and for helping bring the Pan-American Wheelchair Games to Winnipeg that same year.

I was quite honored to be invited with Gene. His two-gold medal winning performance in Heidelberg for winning the discus and pentathlon events, was responsible for him winning the 1972 Lou Marsh Trophy that year. It was the first time that a disabled athlete had won that coveted award. Gene continued winning medals until he retired in 1980. He was a great guy and passed away from a heart attack way too soon.

The hard work that we put in, rewarded us with good results in Belleville. I set personal bests in all my races and best of all, I stopped the clock in the 1500 metre final at 6:52 flat. Graham was happy to say the least, since no-one could find a record of anyone wheeling the 1500 in less than 7 minutes.

This year was the first time any medals were handed out and I was honored to be voted Best Class 2 and Best Male Athlete. But without the benefit of electronic timing, and volunteers manning stopwatches, we still took our winning times with a grain of salt while racing provincially. While I was improving, I knew that everyone else was training as well. Would it be enough?

While I was still riding in a "stock" wheelchair, we had already begun to modify our rides. Most wheelchairs were made to fold for easy transport, and basically consisted of two identical sides held together by a large bolt under the seat. Pull up on the seat and the two sides come together, and the seat folds up. The big problem was that most wheelchairs never completely unfolded, even once you sat in them, and as a result, the back wheels would never be straight up and down. Worse, they would invariably slant out at the top and you were forced to reach over your wheels to grasp the hand-rims. That may not seem like a big difference, but the farther your arms are away from your body, the less power you can generate, and the more stress is put on the joints and muscles.

Our solution to the problem was the invention of the "camber plate", a small piece of flat metal, maybe 2" wide, 3" long and a quarter of an inch thick, with two holes drilled into it. We removed the large bolt from under the seat that held the frame together and then took the "magic" plate and bolted one side of the frame through one of the drilled holes, and did the

Chapter 4: A Taste of Success

same to the other side, so that when you unfolded the chair, your back wheels were now slanted in at the top. You could change the camber of the rear wheels by drilling the holes closer, or farther apart. Now the hand-rims were easier to reach, it was easier to wheel, and the chair had much more stability with the wider wheelbase. And it cornered a lot better than before. The seat sagged in the centre of course, so you either stretched it tight, made new holes and screwed it back to the frame, added a cushion, or had a new seat made.

The front wheels were next on the list for improvements. A wheelchair came with either a pair of 8" spoked front wheels, with thin, solid rubber grey tires, or 5" solid grey plastic wheels with larger balloon tires that had an innertube inside. The spoked wheels fluttered at speed unless they were tightened down, which made cornering more difficult. And while the balloon tires were susceptible to losing air and going flat, they rolled smoother and did not chatter as much. I decided for Winnipeg I would switch to the balloon tire set-up.

The last performance improvement was not mechanical and happened by accident. One of the strange rules at the time was that you could not strap your legs to your chair. You could have a strap behind your legs to stop them from falling off your footplates but a strap to hold them to the frame was not legal. Unfortunately, my legs are too short, and they didn't reach anywhere near the footplates, so when I wheeled quickly, sometimes they would fly off and slow me down.

One day while getting ready to train on the track, I misplaced the running shoes I usually wore, and instead I had to wear my everyday cowboy boots with the big heels. By accident I rested them on the leg strap, and I found that the heels stopped my legs from moving around as much and the added height of my knees prevented me from leaning too far forward and losing my balance. I was also able to generate more power with each push of the chair. Just that small change made me instantly faster. Would my changes be enough to challenge the competition? Not sure. And in the back of my mind, I wondered if resting my feet on the strap would be deemed illegal come race day. I would know soon enough.

With the improvements to my chair, and with a full year of training under Graham's guidance, I felt confident heading into Winnipeg. But I had felt confident before and the results did not materialize. Regardless, the adrenalin was pumping once race day arrived.

In the 100 metres, I got a poor jump at the gun and by the mid-way point, old rival Frank Henderson was beginning to pull away, and I could hear Quebec's Rene Massé gaining on me as well. Frank finished in 21.8, just slightly over his existing record while I held off Rene, and won the silver in 23.2. Faster than my time from Calgary but I was slower than Belleville.

When the 400 rolled around, I put the 100 out of my mind and just focused on the track in front of me and went as hard as I could until I crossed the finish line. I didn't look back and stopped the clock at 1:29.2. Frank was 13 seconds behind, with Kevin Earl of BC winning the bronze. I have a great photo of Frank and I that someone took at the finish line when the race was over. I finally won one, buddy.

I had become the national 400 metre champion with the Canadian record to boot. I was one happy camper, but it was not over. We still had the 1500 metre to wheel. The win would give one of us the bragging rights, for the year at least.

Our 1500 metre Class 2 final was a thrilling race. Frank took off at the opening gun and I had to chase him down and managed to overtake him on the last lap. By finishing in 6:55.8, with Frank crossing in 6:57.7, it meant we both had officially become the first two Canadians to break the 7-minute barrier.

However, during an interview post-race, I ventured the notion that I thought I could go under 5 minutes with better equipment and more top-notch training. It was not received all that well and I was accused of bragging and talking about unrealistic times. We would see.

We had another strong relay team, and we powered our way to the gold and the national title. And for the second year in a row, I ended up with the silver in the slalom.

Meanwhile, over in the pool, Gunther was unbeatable this time, and I came back to Ontario with a silver and two bronze medals. After sweeping my events at the provincials, I had talked myself into thinking this was the year I might swim past him, but I was chewed up and spit out once again. Would I ever learn? My field event career was short-lived, and I was

Chapter 4: A Taste of Success

beginning to think swimming should be the next to go. But we still had to be a multi event athlete, so I carried on.

One medal that was more than satisfying was the bronze we got in basketball. It marked the first time Ontario had won a basketball medal at the nationals, and we were proud of that distinction.

At the Closing Ceremonies, I was over-joyed when it was announced that my 9-medal haul had been enough to have me Voted Best Male Class 2 and Best Male Athlete overall, joining Diane Seeley of BC on the women's side who won for Best Class 2 Female.

Donna Wruth of Manitoba and Ed Batt of Ontario won the Class 1 Best Female / Male awards and Diane Laver of Alberta / Gene Reimer of BC won the Class 3 Awards. Donna was voted Best Female Athlete Overall.

But before we would line up to compete at the Paralympics in Toronto, the classification system would be redesigned once again and expanded to 5 classes. Class 1 would remain the same, but Class 2 was broken down into Classes 2-3, and Class 3 had been replaced by Classes 4-5. Same point system however, and still an equally uncomfortable process.

As a result of the new classification, and after a small debate among our doctors, I was designated a Class 4 athlete. Regardless, this time coming back home to Ontario I felt the games had been successful. Graham's training had obviously made its mark. I was faster and now I felt like I could give the big guys a run for their money.

When I returned to Ontario, I had already decided to leave the Bell and head back to Calgary to see a girl I had met during the nationals in 1972.

During our first volleyball games in Calgary that year, all the guys couldn't help but notice the cute volunteers who were working as line judges during the games. My teammate, John Crawford and I had struck up a conversation with a couple of the girls, and we ended up spending a lot of our free time in their company. John was pretty much smitten, and they did seem to hit it off right away. So much so, that when he got home after the Calgary Games were over, it wasn't that long before he up and packed his bags and moved west. When we caught up with each other in Winnipeg, he talked me into coming out to visit and help get wheelchair sports more established in the Calgary area. With my old buddy Craig riding shotgun, we pack the Ventura to the hilt and headed west a couple of weeks after the team returned home.

And while Craig hitchhiked back to Arthur after a couple of weeks, I stayed with John for the winter, trying my hand at skip tracing and process serving for a lawyer friend of his. But after one Alberta winter under my belt, no real job opportunities and no funds, I was forced to admit defeat and drove back to Ontario in the early spring of '75.

I made my parent's place in Buckhorn my base of operations again when I returned and did the necessary paperwork so I could collect my disability pension for food and gas for the car. Good thing the price of fuel was cheap back then, because I put a lot of miles on the car, going into Toronto and Hamilton, as I tried to reconnect with Graham, Billy and the guys on the basketball team. But it would end up taking a whole year of training before I was able to shed the rust that I had accumulated on my ill-advised trip out west.

Chapter 5:
Starting Over

Since I did no training while out West, it wasn't long after my first wheel back on a track, that I realized how much I was out of shape. Not halfway fit, more like couch potato fit. I would have to get it together if I planned to be in any kind of shape for the Montreal Nationals. Problem was, I still felt down in the dumps. Calgary did not turn out the way I had hoped and coming home alone, my motivational level needed a kickstart.

And as Fate would have it, one of my buddies from Buckhorn spotted me the first day I was back in town, and he took me to a party in Peterborough where I made some new friends. I left feeling that my love life might have taken a turn for the better, but at the very least I was back on home turf as I set my sights on the games in Cambridge.

In April of 1975, American wheelchair racer Bob Hall completed the Boston Marathon to become the first wheelchair athlete in history to wheel that famous race. This would spawn a whole new discipline within wheelchair racing.

The sport of road racing had begun, and in time wheelers would race every distance from the 5K, all the way up to the marathon and beyond. Road racing opened the door to all kinds of innovations since wheeling out on the road was a completely different experience than wheeling on a smooth flat surface with no obstacles to overcome, like there was on a track.

More importantly, the American road racing scene didn't necessarily pay attention to the rules and regulations stated by the Stoke Mandeville Federation, as to what constituted a legal racing chair. The biggest stumbling block in the beginning was the rule that stated the frame had to be made by a recognized wheelchair manufacturing company and had to have four wheels.

Eventually the road racers began to make their own frames. And years later, they formed their own companies and as more athletes around the world did the same, eventually the powers-to-be had no choice but to change the rules. But it was a constant battle that waged for years. Many great racers and road-course record holders never raced at Stoke Mandeville sanctioned games because their chairs would have been deemed illegal.

Americans were racing on the roads long before most of us Canadians took to the pavement, mainly due to the good weather that was found all year round in the southern States and they had almost a decade head-start on us in wheelchair sports in general.

Road racing also gave everyone a look at the machines that their fellow competitors were racing in. As the veterans began to build their own solid-frame chairs, they each had their own idea as to what would work. This allowed other racers a good choice of chairs to choose from when it was time for a new ride. With good weather and the funds to carry it through, a wheeler could travel across America and enter events year-round.

In contrast, in Canada, we had provincial and national games, with a chance to be on the national team if you were good enough, but that was it. There was no road racing, in Ontario at least, until the early '80's.

Up here, we didn't get the chance to check out the varied chairs. You didn't know about new modifications and the upgrades that were available. The evolution of the chair was gaining momentum and unless you were in the right place at the right time, you might pay the price, later down the line. I would learn that the hard way.

In Ontario, 1975 marked the year that the Provincial Wheelchair Games were renamed the Ontario Games for the Disabled, since in our province, the blind and the amputees were just beginning to form their own organizations, and with limited funds, the decision to combine the competitions was made. The TorontOlympiad, scheduled for the following summer was going to be the first international competition in the world with more than one disability being showcased. These Ontario Games were going to be a stepping-stone towards that end.

Chapter 5: Starting Over

This also marked the first year that we received gold, silver and bronze medals for our athletic endeavours, presented by representatives from the newly formed Ontario Wheelchair Sports Association.

While some factions in wheelchair sports were not pleased with the "lumping the disabled together", as athletes it didn't bother us. The more the merrier. We were all trying to persuade society in general, to look past the disability and see the not-so-hidden abilities that we all possessed. In the years that followed, the number of athletes grew in all disability groups. Eventually everyone would have their own championships. Even later in the development of disabled sports, individual sports, like wheelchair tennis, would form alliances with their able-bodied counterparts and become fully integrated. But for now, everyone was invited to the party.

The Ontario Games were held in Cambridge near the end of June, and I managed to win most of my track races. I say most because this year marked the inclusion of the 200 and 800 metre track distances to the race schedule. The 800 had limited entrants, so everyone entered in the event went to the final. No offense to Billy, but when he went by me before we even reached the final straightaway, I realized how much stamina I had partied away out West.

Times were slow, no-one was happy, especially Graham, who vowed to work me "like a rented mule" leading up to the Montreal Nationals. Apparently partying out west for the winter and not playing basketball was not conducive to staying in shape. Graham was glad I was back in the fold, but he knew Montreal would arrive too soon.

And try as I might Montreal was, well, forgettable. Frank ruled the track, and Rene Massé finished not far behind. I won 3 bronze medals. What really ticked me off was brushing a pylon during my slalom run that cost me the gold. I did come home with one gold medal when our Ontario team, consisting of Billy, myself, Bob and Mike O'Brien once again won the 240-metre relay.

It was a poor showing on my part, but I had the rest of the summer and winter's basketball season to get myself back in shape, and in Graham's good graces, so that he could have me peak at the right time. My sights turned to the TorontOlympiad, scheduled for August '76.

That November, I was offered another job with Bell Canada, this time in Centralized Ticket Investigation at Wynford Drive in Scarborough. Fraud investigation was what it amounted to, and I would find out that I enjoyed tracking down individuals who tried to use the phone system illegally.

I got myself another apartment, this time in the Don Mills area, and brought my new girlfriend with me. Life was good! Winter passed quickly, but I still had a lot of work to do.

The media in Toronto, especially the newspapers, had begun to run articles about various athletes that would be competing in Toronto the following year. Even though Montreal was less than satisfactory in terms of results, by the spring, I was asked to do a lot of interviews and I appeared on a few TV shows hyping the upcoming Games.

I was fortunate to work on numerous productions for TV Ontario, a couple of accessibility clips for the St. Lawrence Neighbourhood, plus a featured documentary focusing on my adaptability in life and my racing career. It was produced by good friend, Joan Reid-Olsen of City-TV.

Chapter 6:
First Step Up

In February of '76 I was fortunate enough, as one of a handful of athletes that were expected to do well in the upcoming games in Toronto in August, to be invited to put on a demonstration at the prestigious Toronto Star / Maple Leaf Gardens Indoor Track meet, held in fabled Maple Leaf Gardens.

It was a unique event in many ways. It was advertised on the fact that, for the first time, disabled athletes were being afforded the centre stage along with the likes of the many decorated able-bodied athletes who were in attendance.

Gordie Hope was one of four blind athletes who took turns running an indoor 50 metre race to a packed arena, in total silence. The crowd refrained from making any noise so that the runners could hear their coaches guiding them to the finish line by the sound of their voice. Gordie finished second to Dave Whitehead of Kingston, followed by Toronto's Rico Racini and Bill Shackleton.

I raced against Bob, Mike O'Brien and Billy in the exhibition 50 metre sprint. Mike nipped Bob at the finish line, and I rolled in third. In beating Bob for the first time, Mike made a point of letting the rest of us know that there was going to be a new king of the track from now on. He wasn't happy when I ventured to say that a 50-metre exhibition race proved nothing. The real test would come on the track at the provincials. Then we'd see who was the fastest in Ontario.

What a great experience competing in this meet was though. The crowd was electric, and I hoped it would be as loud when we raced to a packed stadium in Etobicoke during the Paralympics. There was an excellent photo in the Toronto Star the next day, among the results of all the events, of Mike and I racing to the finish line.

The able-bodied athletes that were in attendance certainly had their eyes opened to the possibilities. American Willie Davenport, the 110-metre hurdles gold-medal winner from the '68 Mexico Olympics, was extremely impressed and assured everyone he would be going back to Baton Rouge to make sure "the right people get to hear about this".

Our new apartment was close to a high school track so as soon as the snow melted, I drove over there after work to train. Not the best track though. While it was hard and fast, the occupants of the nearby apartment building had a bad habit of tossing bottles off their balconies to see if they could hit the track. Every day I trained there, there was glass scattered about. Never went on the grass because it was a minefield of busted bottles. So much glass that I got in the habit of keeping a small brush in the trunk of my car, to sweep the track clean before I would train. Last thing I needed was a flat tire.

Going around corners smoothly was always the hardest thing to do while racing in a wheelchair, and one day while training, I found a solution by accident. I was on the track and after a few laps at a good clip, I started to coast. I leaned forward, rested my chest on my knees, grabbed my front forks and steered myself around the corner while I caught my breath. To keep myself coasting I began to push with my right hand but kept steering with my left, and I continued smoothly around the corner. That gave me an idea.

Usually, you had two techniques to choose from to get your chair around the corners. Some athletes simply pushed harder with their right arm while others would bounce the front end of the chair around.

I wheeled onto the straight and pushed as hard as I could down the backstretch. When I reached the corner, I rested on my knees, grabbed the left fork with my hand and pushed as hard as I could on the hand-rim with my right. I flew around the corner, much faster than I had ever gone before, and I was still going full speed when I turned into the straightaway. I might have stumbled onto something here.

I had only been in my new apartment a short time when one of my new Thunderbolt teammates, Marv Murray moved into the building. Marv wasn't

Chapter 6: First Step Up

into racing but being heavily muscled from all the weightlifting he did before he was injured, he was keen to try field events as well as playing basketball with the 'Bolts. It wasn't long before other Thunderbolt teammates joined us and found residence in the building.

Hill climbing is a good workout in your wheelchair, and we had a nice long side-street in front of our building that we could barrel down late at night when there was no traffic to contend with. I loved going wide open down that 1000 metre stretch of road. The workout part began with the push back up the hill, and that took considerable effort, especially after flying down a half-dozen times. Graham wanted me to get into a hill climbing routine because he felt it was a good way for me to build more power. For the three years that I lived there, I spent many hours just speeding down and pushing back up that hill.

Between us and our able-bodied buddies using our extra chairs, there were sometimes five or six of us flying down the road at night. Everyone learned early not to lean too far forward and catch the footplates on the road though, or it was a quick faceplant and an ugly patch of road rash as the reward.

Now that I had a job and a place in Toronto, I didn't have to venture out to Hamilton to meet up with Graham like I did in past years. He had begun to give me a training schedule to follow, and I charted my results and relayed them to him by phone when he called each week. But he told me that when we did get together, I had better be able to duplicate any of the times I had written down. No fudging the books or there'd be hell to pay.

In May there was a big article in the Toronto Star interviewing me as a lead-up to the national championships that were due to take place mid-June at Southwood Secondary school in Cambridge. I talked about the competition we would be up against, and how nice it was to have the other disabilities here with us for the first time. I talked about my technique of steering with one hand around the corners and we touched on the building controversy that surrounded the decision to allow South Africa to send a team to Toronto.

The controversy centered on apartheid, the policy of segregation, and the political, social and economic discrimination against the non-white majority in South Africa that had begun in 1948. While South Africa had been voted into disabled sports the previous year, not all countries believed the team was truly integrated and there were rumours some countries would boycott.

I also had a nice write-up to announce that the Canadian Rehabilitation Council was going to make me a national figure in their advertising campaign. I have a great souvenir of the July 1977 edition of TIME magazine with the full-page Canadian March of Dimes advertisement inside. Included was a cool photo of me taken during the slalom event in Toronto.

The following week we were at the Ontario Games in London. The track was good and hard, and I was looking forward to the competition that the games would bring. When all was said and done, I had gone under my national 100-metre record, set in Winnipeg in '74, while Mike handed Bob his first ever loss, and rewrote the Ontario Class 5 100-metre record.

Mike also wheeled under the national record in the 400 by defeating Bob once again, while I lowered my provincial record. True to his word, Bob retired from racing after these games were over. Mike had become King of the Class 5's. We were set for a 1500-metre showdown.

Back then, at the provincials, the longer 1500 was usually run with the classes combined, since there were not a lot of athletes in every class during the early years. This saved time and made for an exciting race with more athletes in the mix.

The start of the race is not like the sprints, where you have to stay in your lane throughout the race. Internationally, the athlete with the fastest qualifying time gets lane one and the athlete with the next fastest time, lines up to his/her right side. This continues until the entire field is lined up, although if the field was large, you could be lined up behind the first row of racers. Then, at the gun, the usual tactic was to try and get yourself into a comfortable spot along the rail before reaching the bottom of the back stretch. That's when the race starts to get interesting.

With Bob not entered in the 1500, Graham felt that Mike would try and make a statement by taking the lead from the start, so as per his instructions, when Mike bolted into the lead at the sound of the gun, I tucked in behind him as we went down the backstretch for the first time. Graham wanted me to wait until the head of the final stretch to make my move.

Chapter 6: First Step Up

He felt my faster 100-metre time and quicker acceleration would close any gap, and with my one-hand cornering technique, it would set me up nicely for the sprint to the finish.

Back then not everyone understood the significance of *drafting* or tucking in behind the athlete in front of you while wheeling, to cut the wind. In some ways, we felt that being close behind the leader was putting pressure on them to go faster. In the early days you didn't dare get too close to the back wheels, since chairs back then were liable to move around when they got any kind of speed going and that usually caused a crash. Learning to draft was a road racing technique that some of us in Canada didn't learn about, at least not in Ontario until years later.

So, I waited until we came to the final corner, and using my one-hand technique, I accelerated around him and made the final sprint to the finish. He came close but I crossed the line in 6:09 and took 47 seconds off my time from Winnipeg. Bring on the nationals.

All my hard work over the months paid off, and when the dust had settled in Cambridge, and the newly named Canada Games for the Disabled were finished, I felt ready and primed to take on all comers. This had been my best nationals yet.

I set a new national record in the 100 (21.1), a provincial record in the 200, bettered my national 400 metre record and both the 400 and the 1500 were under the existing world records.

My technique of steering my left front wheel of my chair while my right arm powered me through the corners, worked to perfection. The transition from straight-to-corner and corner-to-straight was smooth and I lost no time or momentum trying to correct the chair's natural tendency to roll straight.

I did get serious competition in Cambridge though, most notably from a new athlete from Alberta, by the name of Ron Minor. But I finished 5-0 in my events, including my new favourite, the slalom.

My first-ever gold in the slalom at the nationals was a games' highlight for me, especially since I had to out duel old buddy Frank Henderson and Nova Scotia's great Walter Dann, who won silver and bronze, respectively.

Not to mention that the great American Olympian, Jesse Owens was present and helped hand out medals to a few lucky athletes.

My only silver came in the relay when we were beat by B.C. and that was a strange case. All through the week's competition, BC's Class 5 Pete Colistro had raced on what we thought were illegal 26" rear wheels with larger hand-rims. While much harder to push, you were able to reach higher speeds, and equipped with these big wheels, he dominated his class and re-wrote the 800 and 1500 metre Canadian records. Mike never had a chance.

I asked Graham about the wheels, but no-one had any real answers, so I was kind of left in the dark. Since Pete and I were in different classes, I didn't give it much thought and I should have, but after the nationals, I was riding a great high. The chair was rolling smoothly, and I still had more than a month to fine-tune things, and hopefully peak at the right time. This was not going to be like Germany. I was not coming away empty-handed this time around. Not at home. So, I put the bigger wheels out of my mind.

But if I thought I'd be able to surprise anyone south of the border, that was soon erased when a friend sent me a sports article from the San Francisco Examiner. It was a reprint from a Toronto Star article about the Games, which included my times and an explanation of my one-hand steering technique. Didn't matter. I would be ready. At least I thought so.

As the games in Toronto got closer, and it was officially announced that South Africa was bringing a team of wheelchair, blind and amputee athletes to the TorontOlympiad, the controversy regarding their inclusion began to intensify. Some countries continued to threaten to boycott. The games got a lot of media attention, and a great deal of it was not centered around the up-coming athletic competition.

Sir Ludwig insisted that South Africa had every right to compete because it had fulfilled its obligations and were bringing an integrated team to Toronto.

Suggestions of tokenism were denied by both Sir Ludwig and Canada's Dr. Jackson, and both felt that the presence of South Africa would show progress in eliminating the problem of racial segregation.

It reached a point that Dr. Jackson had to meet the press and explain that the Games would go on, even if the Federal Government continued

Chapter 6: First Step Up

to withhold the $500,000 grant over the question of allowing an integrated South African team to compete.

Dr. Jackson stated that "the ball is in their court, and it's now up to them". There was an outside chance that the Games could have been cancelled or moved to another location, but it ended up being contingent on a decision by the International Stoke Mandeville Games Federation, the governing body for the TorontOlympiad.

"I expect there will be full support for South Africa," said Dr. Jackson. "What might happen is that some nations may boycott the Games. I've received letters from Uganda and Kenya professing their belief that South Africa has broken apartheid (the policy of racial segregation) and deserved to have a team here."

Leading up to the start of the Games I would have been 1 of 60 Canadian athletes, with a total of 1,500 competitors from 47 countries. They were going to be bigger than the Winter Olympics and the largest in the 25-year history of wheelchair sports. At that point, the Games were only rivaled in size by the Summer Olympics and the Commonwealth Games.

Britain and Germany brought the largest team to Toronto. The Soviet Union was sent an invitation, but they didn't admit to having anyone disabled, which was strange at the time, since they were going to be asked to host the 1980 Paralympics.

The Organizing Committee did get a break when the Ontario Jockey Club donated the Woodbine Racetrack for the Opening Ceremonies, thus saving the Committee about $70,000, which would have been the cost to install temporary seating at Centennial Park.

But as the Games got closer, things got progressively worse. Prior to the Opening Ceremonies, Kenya backed out. Yugoslavia pulled its 20-member team and Jamaica withdrew during the Opening Ceremonies.

I took this quote from the Games' opening ceremonies greeting, from Sir Ludwig Guttman, originator of organized sports for the disabled and founder of the Stoke Mandeville Games.

"As the Games have grown bigger, so too have our problems," he said, "but, in the world of the disabled, we are used to overcoming the seemingly insurmountable."

"By remaining firm in our ideals that our world sports movement for the disabled, we must always reject the barrier of race, religion or politics."

However, mere words were not enough, as more teams would withdraw after orders from back home. India withdrew after Poland, Cuba and Hungary pulled their teams. While most teams stayed as spectators, the Hungarian team of 21 and the 38-member Polish team were ordered home immediately.

They all left, except for one Hungarian athlete, Imre Szelenyi, who became the first athlete in the history of the Stoke Mandeville Games to defect. He made a home for himself near the St. Lawrence Market in downtown Toronto.

Sir Guttman was quite emotional himself while addressing the media and said, "We see here a repetition of what happened in Montreal. The feelings of our athletes against the attempts to use our Games as a political pawn is extremely high".

Dr. Jackson said the Games had become "a victim of world-wide publicity about them." "Before, nobody had heard of us, but now that we have been so well-publicized, governments are using them for their own political ends." But they began, nonetheless.

This would have been a great part of the book where I chronicled the demolition of all those who wheeled against me that week. Success after all the hard work and dedication. I felt confident in predicting gold in at least the 800 metre and perhaps more. But the first day on the track and after my first glimpse of the competition, I realized it was not going to happen.

Started out well enough. Weather was nice, the track was dry. The team got on the track early, to warm up and to get used to the artificial surface that covered the Centennial track in Etobicoke.

I had a couple of laps in me, when suddenly a pack of wheelies went rolling by and down the backstretch. Mostly Americans, but a couple of European athletes as well. All using 26" wheels. What the hell was going on? And not only that, but some of these oversized wheels sported much smaller diameter hand-rims, which I had never seen before.

Now the rationale behind the changes certainly made sense. The 26" wheel gives you an advantage over the 24" version since you cover more

Chapter 6: First Step Up

ground per stroke. On the other hand, you need extra strength to get it rolling and to maintain the speed.

The smaller hand-rims give you an extra gear because you can shift down to them once you get rolling by pushing off your tires. Again, they require more strength, but you can achieve a higher top end speed.

You can bet I wasn't a happy camper that morning, as I soon realized that come race day, if things stayed the same, I'd be hard pressed to win a medal of any colour.

After talking to Graham, my worst fears were realized. There was talk that all chairs were to be deemed legal for this competition, and afterwards the Stoke Mandeville Federation would come up with a new set of rules and guidelines regarding all equipment, and would in fact, also tweak the disability classes once more, in another attempt to level out the playing field before the '80 Holland Paralympics.

It became obvious from talking to some of the other racers, that the reason that Pete knew about the big wheels, was because the BC athletes had an opportunity to train down south in the winter. California boasted great weather with lots of room for athletes to wheel, and going down there, Pete had a front row seat to all the new ideas and equipment improvements that came from south of the border. He knew that the Americans were coming north with the big wheels and small hand-rim combination, a concept credited to great American Hall of Fame racer Gary Kerr. Pete came prepared to Toronto. The rest of us were left in the dark.

The big wheel / small hand-rim made great sense, a stroke of genius if you ask me, but why didn't the rest of us know about this? Especially after the nationals. Did our officials think the rest of us could still win, regardless of the disadvantage? Were they hoping the wheels would be deemed illegal? Unlikely since they would not have allowed Pete to wheel with them at the nationals. We waited for a ruling from Stoke Mandeville about what was and was not legal. The rest of us were clearly up against the wall here.

The end of the debate happened after Graham had returned from the Rules Committee meeting, held to let the countries know where things stood.

It was rumoured that the Americans threatened to pull the team if they couldn't wheel with the chairs they brought. With so many countries pulling their teams because of the inclusion of a South African team, the games could not afford to have such a large contingent of athletes withdraw.

Besides, it was argued, if the rules are going to be looked at after this competition, why not highlight the advantages that the new equipment brings to the sport? With some European countries having entered racers using the big wheels as well, it was decided. All bets are off. Race what you brought. I had to scramble and decide what my next plan of attack would be.

I went to E & J with my dilemma, and they said they would do what they could to put together a big wheel / small hand-rim combination for me. Whether they could finish them before the games were over, remained to be seen, because they had regular work to do, and the company had a pit-crew that was servicing all the chairs during the Olympiad. I knew they would try though.

But from the first day of actual competition, it was as I feared. The big wheel / small hand-rim combination proved to be deadly. If you were wheeling on 24's, you were fighting for scraps unless the competitors in your class were wheeling on the small wheels as well.

At this point in our sports history, not all disability classes raced the same number of events, nor were they allowed to race all the distances offered. In Toronto, every class raced the 100, but the newly included 200 was confined to Class 2 and 3 athletes.

All classes raced the 400 but only the Class 4 and 5 athletes wheeled the 800. The 1500 was also restricted to just the Class 4 and 5 competitors.

The 100 metre finals were a true indication of just how powerful and dominant the US track team was during this competition. Of the 12 medals up for grabs, the Americans took home half of the haul. Class 2 Gary Kerr, Class 3 Jim Hernandez, and Class 4 Dave Kiley, all won gold. Charlie Williams took bronze in the Class 3 100 and Ray Lewandowski took silver in Class 4. Rolf Johannon of Sweden was the only athlete outside of America to win gold, defeating Randy Wix in the Class 5 100 metre final.

One slip on my hand-rim during my Class 4 semi-final cost me the chance to make the top eight. In the final, American Dave Kiley wheeled a 19.4 and set a new Class 4 100-metre Paralympic record that earned him the gold medal.

Chapter 6: First Step Up

In the Class 2 200 final, places were reversed as Kerr was not able to hold off Eusebio Valdez of Mexico like he had in the 100. However, Americans' Jim Hernandez and Charlie Williams went one two for the US in the Class 3 final.

The US was shut out in the Class 2 400, with Valdez picking up his 2nd gold, but the Class 3 final saw Charlie Williams of the US pick up his first gold with teammate Jim Hernandez winning the bronze.

I made the final for the Class 4 800, and I was super nervous at the starting line. Graham had been studying the competition all week once he realized what we were up against, in hopes he could come up with a game plan to combat the disadvantage that the big wheels presented.

We had hoped that in the sprint races, the 24" wheels would enable us to get a quicker jump at the gun and get to the finish before the big wheels started rolling. But the results proved otherwise. If you were already used to the big wheels and started off by pushing on your tires or the top of your spokes to initiate movement, there was not much of a difference to be gained and once they were rolling, they pulled away.

Now that we were preparing to roll longer distances, Graham sat me down and told me it was time to be realistic. Regardless of the plans we had going in, which was to take the lead and not look back, the reality of the situation meant we had to rethink our strategy. He felt it better to let others take the lead, and then work myself into a position for a later kick that might get me into the medals.

Come race day I was lined up in a middle lane, and at the gun we all took off. Down the backstretch we went, and by the time we merged at the top of the straight I had passed two athletes.

A quick glance showed me that the two front-runners were dueling each other for the lead and had created a gap between them and a string of three other racers, as we continued down the track.

The group of three were beginning to spread out when I began to pick up my pace. I passed one competitor as we came out of the first corner on the bell lap and chased down another wheeler as we went down the backstretch. Coming up to the final corner I had a full head of steam and was gaining on the third-place athlete as we rounded the bend.

Since he had the inside lane blocked in front of me, it was my intention to go around him once we were on the straightaway, where I would have some room to manoeuvre. However sometimes racers like to move away from the inside. More than one athlete has clipped the inside rail of a track during games past and crashed. Moving out gives you a bit of a cushion if your chair moves around, but it provided an opportunity for me. When he moved farther towards the middle of the track, I took the straight line and darted between him and the rail.

Once I passed him, I knew he didn't have a finishing kick and I wasn't going to be caught. In a blink it seemed, I had crossed the line and won the bronze. Not the colour I was hoping for, and not the colour I had foolishly promised, but it was my first Paralympic medal, and I did it on 24" wheels.

As expected, US racer Dave Kiley won the gold in a battle with Remi Van Ophen of the Netherlands. I have a great picture from the newspaper of him flying around the corner, using my one-handed cornering technique! You're welcome, Dave.

But in the Class 5 final, Pete was primed and ready to give them a run for their money. No doubt wearing the Canadian singlet must have given him a great sense of pride when he won the Class 5 800 over American Randy Wix, on his way to winning Canada's only track gold medal of those Paralympics.

Soon it was time for the 1500. During my heat, I was able to lower the existing world record down to 5:35.0, and I had the opportunity to help a fellow racer as well.

I led my heat from start to finish and a few of us lapped an athlete from Colombia during the race. After I crossed the finish line, I coasted around the corner and caught up to the Colombia athlete who was still struggling down the backstretch. I moved over to an outside lane but continued to pace him, telling him to keep going as hard as he could as we wheeled towards the final corner.

I wheeled with him around the first half of the corner, and with a few last words of encouragement I stopped and let him wheel down the straight to the finish line.

Beforehand, after I had crossed the finish line, the crowd had gone silent when they had realized the Colombian racer was not going to stop, even though the race was over. But as he began to push the final stretch, the crowd finally erupted and cheered like mad until he crossed the finish line.

The people in the stands learned a good lesson from that race. The disabled do not quit, regardless of the circumstances. I felt good that I helped him along.

Between then and the final, a representative from E & J showed up with a big wheel/small hand-rim combination for me to try out. John Aldredge had become a good friend from the first time I ventured into E & J years ago and he worked hard to give me a chance at least.

The wheels were heavier, and they did take a lot more effort per stroke than I was used to. My hand-rims had shrunk from the usual 22" diameter to 16". They would have to do. I was desperate and thought it was my best chance to medal.

Graham did not think it was a good idea because I hadn't had much time to get accustomed to them except for a few laps when they arrived. Part of my success is my power to weight ratio. I was light and so was my chair. I was able to get away with less strokes and more glide and this enabled me to stay with athletes who possessed considerably more power. Could I pull it off with heavier wheels and the smaller push-rims? We would see soon enough.

By the time I lined up for the 1500 final, we had already planned to follow the same strategy as I employed in the 800. Let the leaders go out, pull in behind someone and wait for an opportunity.

I stayed as close as I could, but by the end of the first lap, I realized I could not keep their pace on these new wheels for the whole race, regardless of my high fitness level. I hoped I would still have a finishing kick.

In the end, the three medalists rolled away from the rest of the field, and although my finishing burst was enough to go around the rest, it was only good for a distant 4th.

True to form, American Dave Kiley won the Class 4 1500, setting a record of 5:32 ahead of Mexican Rene Corona and Birger North of Sweden. The winning time was what made me start to second guess my decision to use the big wheels. If I had stayed with my regular set-up, I think I would have given them a run for their money. I had no way of knowing but the thought ticked me off regardless.

Pete battled all the way in his Class 5 final, and he was just beaten to the wire for gold by American Randy Wix. That made it one each.

While my track results were not at all what I had hoped for, I was still looking forward to the slalom competition. Being the new Canadian champion for less than a month, I was eager to see how well I could do against the stiffest competition possible.

In the early days, if you competed in the slalom, you usually competed in your basketball chair, but after these Games were over, and I got a glimpse of what I thought were slalom chairs, I had decided that I wanted to build a slalom chair for competition.

First thing I noticed was the number of competitors, both male and female that were entered in the slalom. It easily rivaled the number of athletes that usually compete for the 100-metre crown. It took more than an hour for each athlete from every class, to race through the course.

As usual, with no heats to go through, competitors in each class drew starting numbers out of a hat, and once you made your run, you sat there, and waited. And watched each athlete as he navigated the course, while trying to calculate their estimated time in your head.

Most prominent were the Japanese, and they dominated most of the classes. I was told that in Japan the slalom was the highlight event of their National Games for the Disabled.

And while it looked as if all their small chairs were built for just this event, their coach had a simple answer: small people = small chairs. And their skill level was immediately evident in all the Class finals.

In my Class, Japan's Hoshi Yoshiteru blazed through the course in 1:01.7 for an easy gold medal, while Brian McNicoll of New Zealand and I battled for the silver/bronze. Brian came away with the silver in a time of 1:11.0 and I took bronze, finishing in 1:12.7. The difference was my brush of a gate during my run that cost me the dreaded 3 second penalty. Still, the result made me a little happier considering the bronze in the 800 was my only hardware to that point. I was beginning to enjoy the slalom more and more.

Yoshiteru's teammate Masami Morimoto won gold in the women's Class 5 event finishing over 14 seconds faster than Canadian Joanne McDonald of

Chapter 6: First Step Up

Newfoundland who took home silver. But Joanne was just getting warmed up, her eventual Hall of Fame career would unfold as the years went on.

In the slalom for quad competitors, good buddy Ed Batt of St. Catherine's took home bronze in the Class 1A event.

With the two bronze medals in my pocket, I was happy to a certain extent. At least I had contributed a couple of medals towards Canada's total haul. I had something to show for my efforts and I didn't finish the competition empty handed like I did in Germany, but a little ticked off with the way the racing competition went. I vowed to myself that I'd be fully armed for the next showdown.

Team wise, I thought we did well. We ended up 6th in the world, with 25 gold, 30 silver and 31 bronze.

The track team accounted for a gold - 2 silver and 3 bronze. It was ok, but as a team, we were getting faster and deeper as our talent pool continued to grow. One day I would look back and realize that this was the start of a steady stream of world-class Canadian racers that would make their mark on the world stage for decades to come. That included my new Canadian teammate, Ron Minor, who had mentioned to me while he was in Toronto that the nationals were going to be in his hometown of Edmonton the next summer, and that he had sights on my Canadian records. Not already, I've just gotten used to having them!

That winter heralded another steppingstone in the advancement of wheelchair basketball in Ontario. By now the Thunderbolts had players from all over Ontario who played on the team, and a good number of them travelled more than a few miles to come to practice and to go to our away games south of the border.

In the summer, more than a few players had stated their desire to start a team in their hometown and form a small league for players around the southern part of the province.

This resulted in the formation of the Southern Ontario Wheelchair Basketball League. The SOWBL began with 5 teams, the London Forest City Flyers, headed by future NWBA Hall of Fame player, Bruce Russell… the Kitchener Twin City Spinners, formed by two Lakewood Camp buddies,

Dean Mellway and Al Slater, and the St. Catharines Charioteers, a team that boasted fellow Paralympian Ed Batt.

The rest of the Toronto area players assumed that they would form an SOWBL team, as well as keep the Thunderbolts going. However, unknown to some, there was a handful of players that wanted to break away and form another organization altogether.

The result was that while the Thunderbolts continued playing in the NWBA, we had two Toronto teams for the start of that first SOWBL season. The Toronto Spitfires were formed by fellow racer Mike Bryce and his brother Bob and close friend Jerry Tonello. Flo Aukema was their starting centre.

The remaining players, including original Thunderbolt Dale Moe, gathered the rest of the players together and pointed out that if we wanted to play ball, we'd have to form another team. We decided to call ourselves the Toronto Golden Wheels and prepared for our first season.

It wasn't long before we realized that despite our best intentions, there were teams that didn't have enough players for a starting lineup. The solution was to allow an able-bodied player to fill in until the team found another disabled player. In time, many felt that this decision had opened Pandora's Box, never to be closed again.

Chapter 7: Redemption

Once the Paralympics were over, I continued to use the big wheel/small hand-rim set-up that E & J had built for me, until snow brought outdoor training to a stop. It took me until the end of the summer to get used to them, though. They were a lot harder to push than what I had been accustomed to, and by the end of the summer, I decided that not only did I want better back wheels and different sized hand-rims, but I wanted to have a new racer built.

Toronto had convinced me that I needed a new racing chair that would solve the problem of my legs moving around and coming off the leg strap, and a chair that was made for the big wheel/small hand-rim combination. Now that I had a job again, I felt I could afford the expense. I went to Everest & Jennings again to see if they would build me a custom chair to my specifications.

In a regular chair, the footplates are down near the ground so a person's legs can be fully extended to be comfortable. But, as I said, my legs are short, and while we were allowed a strap behind them to prevent them from falling off, we were still not allowed to tie them down. While having my feet resting on the strap helped, it didn't prevent them from moving around and that was still enough to throw off my balance.

To prevent this from happening, I intended to have the chair made with the footplates high enough that my feet would rest on them properly and the plates welded on an angle that would keep my feet flat and fully supported. While I couldn't strap my feet down, with the heels of my cowboy boots wedged against the back of the footplates, it would ensure that my legs did not move. The slanted footplates would keep my knees just high enough that I could lean forward without losing my balance. And I wanted it on the smallest kid's frame that I could squeeze into, making it as tight as possible. I was hoping to replicate the feeling I had as a kid racing around in that tiny Johnson & Johnson chair at Lakewood Camp.

While the chair was being built, I began to look around for better rear wheels to attach to the new hand-rims I was having made. I went to a local bike store to see what they had to offer. It didn't take long before they found me a set of rims that were considerably lighter and thinner, and they matched them with a pair of high-pressure sew-up tires with much less tread. Holding the new wheel in one hand and the old one in the other proved to me that they were going to help going forward. There was a big weight difference. I went back to E & J with the new wheels and tires and had them build me a new pair of 14" hand-rims.

I had been using the grey balloon tire set-up on the front end of my chair since before the Winnipeg Nationals in '74, and while they worked better under speed, they did not roll nearly as long or freely as did the spoked wheel set-up. I wondered if there were better bearings in the spoked wheel.

I removed the balloon wheels from the forks to get a better look and realized they had a plastic dust cap over the opening, to prevent debris from getting inside and seizing the bearings up. I took an X-Acto knife and cut away the dust guards and found that both sets of wheels were using the exact same bearings, but when I spun the wheel, it rolled a good minute longer than the one with the guard. This was a little trick that I hoped would make a big difference.

I knew without the plastic guards, the bearings were going to get full of junk, so my idea was to flush them with WD-40 before each race to keep them clear.

Then I turned my attention to my back wheels. I was happy with the improvement that the new wheels and smaller hand-rims would provide, but could I find better bearings than what the regular E & J wheelchair hubs came with?

I tracked down a company that made bearings in hopes of finding some of better quality, and when I did, I took a wheel with me to the SKF factory

Chapter 7: Redemption

in Scarborough to try my luck. I told them I wanted them for a racing wheelchair, and did they have bearings that would fit this hub?

They were quite keen to help me out and when they saw the original bearings that were in the hub, they smiled and said they were sure they had something much superior in stock to replace the originals.

They did indeed have better bearings, much better actually, and I was a happy camper leaving the facility with a free bag full of bearings that would keep me going for years to come.

In the meantime, as well as all the interval training on the track, I continued to climb that hill outside the apartment building again and again. Eventually, I got in the habit of trying to see what kind of top speed I could hit while going down without touching my wheels. I didn't know then, but in later years, my willingness to go full speed down any hill regardless of the incline, without trying to slow down, would keep me competitive in certain events once I began racing on the road. In all the years I raced, I never crashed once in competition, though it was on a scary training run that made up my mind to go wide open in the first place.

One of my new Thunderbolt teammates that had moved into the building where I lived, was Brien Foran. Going into the hospital for a routine operation, complications left him confined to a wheelchair when a blood clot was not found in time. Once out of the hospital at Lyndhurst, he was keen on playing basketball and joined the Thunderbolts. Now he wanted to try racing.

So, one evening, we went out wheeling together. I picked a road I had travelled on by car, but it was the first time I had decided to train along this stretch in my chair. I knew there was a downhill section, but I guess my perspective of the decline was not that accurate.

As we began our descent, I realized it was a lot steeper and longer than I remembered. I had just begun experimenting with padding my handrims, and I obviously did a poor job, because when I realized how fast I was travelling, I tried to slow down. But when I grabbed the rims, the tape and the foam padding that I had added, began to unravel. I tried to use my hands to slow down, but they heated up so quickly I ended up friction burning both my index fingers. All I could do was reach down into my tuck and use my hands to steer the front wheels to make sure I was at least rolling straight.

I flew down that hill at breakneck speed and although I love to go fast, it scared the crap out of yours truly. At one point, a car pulled up along side of me, but either backed off, or I left him behind, because I beat him to the stoplights that luckily were far enough past the bottom of the hill that I could slow down safely. Once we stopped, the driver rolled down his window and said I was going over 60 miles per hour! Said I scared the life out of him. Me too, buddy, me too!

Brien was amazed at the speed I reached but said I was lucky I didn't hit something on the road or that would have been all she wrote. He was right of course. The wheelbase on the chairs we used back then were short, and all you had to do was lean too far forward or hit a pebble with those small front wheels, and you were going for a tumble.

Back home, relaxing on the couch with a beer, I realized how much of an advantage that gave me over Brien on that section. Being a lot heavier than me, he would have travelled a lot faster and a lot farther if he had just "let 'er go", but wisely chose otherwise.

Years later, I got in the habit of using my "tuck and roll" method, if you will, to either make up ground or to pass as many competitors as I could. I realized there were only a hand-full of racers willing to fly down a steep incline without controlling their speed to some extent. And while I can't say the technique was the difference between winning or losing, it did enable me to shave time off the clock that I wouldn't have been able to do otherwise, and sometimes helped me move up in the standings.

The first time I rolled onto the track and began wheeling in my new chair, I got excited. The chair fit perfect, my legs were situated exactly where I had wanted them, and I flew around the corner with one hand like I had never done before. I was looking forward to my first test.

I had my new chair for a couple of weeks when I had the opportunity to test it out in an actual race before the provincials. Thanks to Graham, an exhibition 400 metre race was added to the Ontario Masters Track & Field Championships in June. They were held at McMaster University, a week

Chapter 7: Redemption

before the Brantford Ontario Games were about to start. Brien and Billy and I were going to wheel against each other before a packed stadium.

I was pumped for the opportunity because I wanted an idea of how my training was going, before I lined up to compete in Brantford, and I wanted to gauge how much the chair would help going forward.

The McMaster track was good and hard, there was no wind, and it was nice and warm outside. I knew going in that the world record was 1:28.6 and although I didn't know for sure who had set that record or when, I wanted to get as close to it as I could. Graham intended to have this exhibition race done by the book, with the same timekeepers as the able-bodied runners used, so that if I did manage to set a record, it would be officially recognized.

While Billy and Brien gave me a good run for my money, I put my head down and pushed for all I was worth. The look on Graham's face was all I needed to know that I was heading in the right direction, but I was pleasantly surprised to find that I had stopped the clock at 1:16.8. Thanks to Graham's effort, it became a recognized national record and well under the existing world mark. One down on my personal list.

Success in the exhibition 400 had me looking forward to wheeling in Brantford, and my competition with Mike would see another chapter in our battle for provincial bragging rights.

My Canadian Class 4 record in the 100 was 21.1 and a far cry from American Dave Kiley's time of 19.4, set last year, but I was satisfied when I stopped the clock at 19.8 in my final. Perhaps in Edmonton, if the conditions are ideal and the competition was as tough as I thought it would be, I might have a chance at breaking the record.

I didn't quite duplicate my record time from the Master's in my 400 final, but I stopped the clock at 1:18.3. And again, I hoped that stiffer competition would help to get it lowered when I headed out west in August.

I added a win in the 800 and that left the 1500 to contest. As usual, all the classes would race together, and that set Mike and I up for another showdown.

By now he owned all the Class 5 provincial records and was significantly quicker than when we raced at the provincials the year before. Like me, he had received the same Fate as I did against the 26" wheels in Toronto, and in the meantime, he had modified his chair to work with the big wheels, had his own coach, and was looking for better results this year.

At the gun, he took the lead and when I attempted to go around him down the backstretch, he picked up his pace. It was apparent that he intended to stay there and not let me pass. We still did not recognize the advantage that drafting would have over time, since we were still not racing on the road like the Americans had been doing for years, and Mike was focused on leaving me behind. So, I tucked up behind him once we hit the bottom of the backstretch and kept enough distance to prevent us from touching wheels until I waited to make my move.

Going wide open, I put a lot of strokes on my hand-rims when needed, but because I was so light, most of the time I liked to take longer strokes and then glide a bit before taking another push.

In the 1500, if I found an athlete in front of me, I tried to take one push for every two of theirs and just readied myself to pick up the pace, if the opportunity presented itself.

On the bell lap of this race, Graham was standing nearby on the infield, and he yelled at me to go around him. But I hesitated to do it so early and stayed where I was.

Instead, I went out and around him at the bottom of the backstretch under a full head of steam, using my one-hand technique to propel me around the corner. Once on the straight, I put my head down and gave it all I had. I clocked 5:05.0, well under the 5:32.0 world record.

But if I had gone when Graham had told me to go, would I have cracked the 5-minute 1500-metre barrier like I said was possible, a few years before? Not sure, but while I would eventually roll under the 5-minute mark, the distinction of being first was destined to fall to a fellow Canadian the following year.

Not a lot of work was left to do leading up to Edmonton for what was now named the Canadian Games for the Physically Disabled, but one thing I did want to do was spruce-up my chair before heading west. I planned on putting on a show, regardless of who I went against. I made no predictions leading up to the nationals though. I would never make that mistake in my career again. But I still had to have some fun.

Chapter 7: Redemption

First thing I did was take the chair completely apart. Instead of plain chrome I wanted something flashier. It was time to "Pimp my Ride".

With help from the guys, I spray-painted the whole frame metal-flake red. Once it was dry, the hard part began. Earlier, I had bought a couple of rolls of a product called "diffraction" tape. Sometimes called prism tape, it's made to reflect light and send a rainbow of colors in all directions. It was perfect for what I had in mind.

We went about measuring every straight piece of tubing, cutting the tape to size, and then carefully applying it until the chair was completely covered except the sections where the frame had been welded together. Reassembled, it was a moving light show. Together with the black t-shirt I had made that said "Smokin Stoddart" across the back, I was ready to race. Didn't care if I reminded someone of *Kramer* from the old Seinfeld show, wearing his "Coat of Many Colours". I went to Edmonton meaning business.

Unfortunately, Fate showed its face once more when my home life came apart a couple of weeks before I was to leave for Edmonton. My girlfriend announced that she was homesick. Since she hadn't found a job yet, she was bored with staying in the apartment all day while I went to work. Plus, she hated the big city and decided she was moving back home to be closer to her family. I headed west angry and with a heavy heart.

For the first time in the history of our sport, these Canadian Games for the Disabled included the blind and the amputee athletes, but again, not everyone was happy. There were those who went on record saying that the Canadian Wheelchair Sports Association had all the experience and had been running the show for years, not to mention footing the bill as well. Why should they help pay for another group's participation? Money spent on other groups meant less funds for CWSA.

As well, because there were different groups of disabled athletes, the press had been calling us "wheelchair athletes" or "blind athletes" to make the distinction. There were those in the Association that thought people were getting used to saying just "athlete" when referring to wheelchair athletes and they thought it was a step in the wrong direction.

Ontario had already proven that the combination had merit from an athletic point-of-view, from the reactions following our provincials. Everyone likes sports and the unique difficulties presented by each group, just further showed that a person could overcome a lot and still do a lot, regardless of the type of handicap they were faced with.

Over the years, each organization would expand and by the early '80's, the cerebral palsied athlete would be recognized, and they would eventually have their own games, as disabled sports continued to expand.

To my surprise, when I arrived in Edmonton the local newspapers were already talking about a showdown between hometown racer Ron Minor and myself. There were a lot of articles in the Edmonton newspapers that week, promoting the games and promising exciting races in the days to come. Every day that the games were on, the results and highlights from the day before could be found in the Sports section. If only the weather had co-operated.

Because of the rain that would ultimately fall nearly every day, the Opening Ceremonies were held inside. Looking at all the overhead lights inside the arena gave me a great idea. I rode in my new chair for the Opening Ceremonies instead of my basketball chair and the lights inside the area sent out rainbows of colour off my racer whenever I moved. Wheeling around the arena was great fun. I looked like a rolling Disco ball. But all flash and no substance? We'll see.

While the rain came down relentlessly all week, and the stands were virtually empty, it didn't prevent us from rewriting the record book though.

On the track there were numerous races in all the Classes that went down to the wire, and as the years had progressed, more and more competitors in all classes arrived to give it their best. Not only did I face the challenge that Alberta's Ron Minor presented, but a half dozen other athletes from other provinces, were intent on winning as well.

One of my goals leading into the year was to erase the existing 100 metre record of 19.4 that was set by US gold medal winner Dave Kiley in Toronto the year before. While I got closer at the provincials in Ontario, I wanted to go even faster in Edmonton.

It was one of the rare races that didn't have the rain pouring down that week and that helped my cause considerably. It was a battle down the whole length of the track, but I held off the field to win in 18.35. It was a new Canadian record and under the existing world record. Ron and Frank Henderson took silver and bronze, respectively. One down, five more to go.

Chapter 7: Redemption

Throughout the week, it was a continuous battle at every distance. Using my one-hand cornering technique, I wheeled a 1:17.81 in the 400 final for the gold, and while I had hoped to improve on my time from the exhibition race in Ontario, the conditions were not the best.

Not everything went my way however as I was the creator of my own downfall in the 200 final. The use of my one-hand cornering technique enabled me to go around corners with a smooth transition from the straightaway into the corner and back out again, but it didn't dawn on me that it only worked efficiently under a full head of steam.

I had only wheeled the 200 a couple of times since it was a new event, so when the gun sounded at the start, I only took a few two-handed pushes, before I switched to pushing with my right hand and steering with my left. The lag in time that it took to get up to full speed was more than enough for the competition. This time it was Ron who jumped out in front, and with a good lead, I couldn't reel him in. He clocked in at a new Canadian record time of 38.88, to my 38.90. Lesson learned.

The Class 4 world 800 record was 2:47 flat, also owned by American Dave Kiley, and it was next on my list. While it was cold the day of the race, there was only a smattering of rain and hardly any wind when we lined up.

Thankfully, because I learned to hate wind. Even though I always remembered my old teammate Bob Simpson's words about not letting the conditions affect your performance, wind caused more havoc with my ability to wheel in a straight line, or push into a headwind, during my career than any other factor. The price for being light, I guess.

My strategy was to go out hard at the beginning and let the field try and catch me, both in this the 800, and in the longer 1500. I always watched who was close behind me and if I thought they were coasting, my strategy was not to pick up the pace, but to slow it down slightly. If they didn't make a move to pass, I kept that pace and conserved my energy. But I would bolt for home the moment I felt someone trying to overtake me. Early on, or later in the race, I would not let you pass me if I could help it. If I couldn't hold you off, too bad for me but I liked rolling out in front if I could.

I took the lead as the pack converged and didn't look back. I'm not sure who came second or third, to tell the truth, but I was satisfied with a

2:43.78 time, and it shaved a couple of seconds off the record. It left only the 1500 and the slalom on my personal list.

Being at the nationals, there were enough competitors in each class, so there was more than one 1500 final to be contested. Our Class 4 race would not be combined with the Class 5 final, as it was during our provincials.

As I mentioned earlier, rain had begun on the first day of competition and it was no different during this race. It was coming down hard and getting a grip on the hand-rims was proving difficult for everyone.

At the gun, Ron surged out in front of the pack, with me close behind. I followed him around the bend and stayed back just far enough so I didn't clip wheels as we raced, and so that the water that was coming off his rear wheels didn't reach me.

I realized early in the race that, because of the conditions, the pace was much slower than what Mike had set when we raced in the hot sun at our provincials. There was not going to be an opportunity to better the 5:05 I set under ideal conditions in Ontario. This was going to be a race of strategy. So, I continued to tuck in behind, and waited. No-one else in the field made a move behind me, so my thought was that, once we reached the final corner, I would try and go around him.

We stayed this way down the final backstretch, and with a full head of steam, I went out and around on the corner and headed for home and the win, stopping the clock in 6:11.

Graham was happy with my outcome, because unknown to either Ron or I, he had a secret bet going on with Ron's older brother, who had come down out of the stands to vouch for Ron and to "fire one across the bow", so to speak.

It was all in fun though. Ron and I were team-mates on more than one occasion throughout our careers and we always managed to have a good time while we were away. We would only race against each other once more though, before another reclassification would see us in different Classes for the rest of our careers.

In the Class 5 1500 final, Mike pulled away from Kevin Earl of Edmonton to win the gold with a new Canadian record of 5:43.0. A new racer from Newfoundland, by the name of Mel Fitzgerald won the bronze. The "Newfie Bullet" had arrived.

Chapter 7: Redemption

The last event on the track was the 4x100 metre relay. This was the first year that the relay became a recognized event and followed the same format that the able-bodied used. Our Ontario team consisted of veteran Ron Thompson, Mike, me, and young rookie John Urocioli. John had sprinted to a gold medal in the Class 5 200 final and with the new blood on the team, we led from start to finish and added the relay crown to Ontario's medal haul.

All that was left was my new favourite race: the slalom, and for all his size, Ron could really move through the gates. He was as tough on the obstacle course as he was on the track. This was true for Frank Henderson as well since he had been National slalom champion in Games past, as had another competitor who was entered, Steven Little of N.B. This was going to be a battle.

Having won the slalom event the year before and capping it off with a Paralympic bronze in Toronto, I felt like I was the guy to beat going into the competition. But I knew past success counts for nothing, I couldn't afford to incur any penalties if I wished to defend my title.

An Edmonton newspaper article printed earlier in the week had already set the stage for a slalom showdown, and fortunately for me, I wheeled a penalty-free race like I did in the unexpected previous day's preliminary round. That was the ticket to capture the gold.

A lot of great athletes put on quite a show in Edmonton and I was honored to be named Best Class 4 Athlete and Overall Male Athlete for the second time in my career.

But as great as my track success felt, the one medal that I helped win off the track was equally satisfying. Ever since the games had begun in '67, Ontario had never won a gold medal in wheelchair basketball. The closest we came was the bronze we won in Winnipeg in '74. But we had a good team in '77. Maybe not the best, but we were looking for a medal regardless.

Perennial powerhouse BC had been going against any one of the western provinces in the final game since Canada began playing interprovincial basketball. That year was expected to be no different.

During the round-robin Alberta beat Manitoba and BC beat Nova Scotia. We beat Saskatchewan and won by default over Newfoundland who didn't have enough players. We lost by a good margin against BC, but that was expected.

In the semi-final, we played our best defensive game of the tournament and stymied their great captain Reg McClellan, Ron, and his Edmonton teammates to make the gold medal game.

The second game, on paper at least, had BC gunning for another title if they got past Manitoba. We had a tough time against BC during the round-robin part of the Championship but with at least a silver medal as our reward for making the final, we hoped to give either team a run for their money, with no pressure on us.

This semi-final was a real thriller and ended with Manitoba captain, the late great John Lundie, dropping a Seth Curry-like 3-ball from way deep in the corner with time running out, that shocked the BC squad and allowed Manitoba to escaped with a 36-35 upset win. Greatest, longest, most important clutch wheelchair basketball shot I ever saw in my 15 years of playing ball. Sweet. A moment and a great athlete to remember forever.

It made the final game historic since it was the first time in 10 years that British Columbia was not represented in the Final. With virtually the whole BC provincial team made up of players from the NWBA West Coast division Vancouver Cable Cars, they were always a formidable group. The final was also historic in that it was the first time in 9 years that Manitoba was battling for gold. An Ontario team had never reached the Finals.

In the gold medal game, our defense, anchored by our big men Flo Aukema and Bruce Russell shut down Manitoba's inside game. Combined with the success of our fast break, we managed to squeak out the win, and being a part of the first ever Ontario team to be crowned National Champions was a satisfying achievement.

With 4 new Canadian records, pending world records and the slalom crown, I was a happy camper heading home. But once I got there, I knew I was going to face an empty apartment and the realization that I was alone again. The guys were there, of course. Living in the same building meant there was always someone to hang around with, but partying was not as much fun as it should have been.

Near the end of August, I received an invitation to a competition in Quebec. The invitation was from then Mayor Jean Corbeil of Ville d' Anjou which read:

Chapter 7: Redemption

"My community has decided to offer to the elite amongst the best Canadian wheelchair athletes, a unique opportunity to compete in a very selective competition that will be held in Anjou, Quebec on September 23rd, 24th, and 25th, 1977. It shall be known as the Anjou Super Challenge and will be restricted to the top 50 Canadian wheelchair athletes who will be invited to match their skills on a personal basis".

I was super excited. What an honour to get picked and while I knew the competition format was essentially a pentathlon, and I would be at a disadvantage, there was no way I was going to turn down this invitation. Though I hadn't had the heart to train since I got back from Edmonton, it got me out of the apartment.

The competition was held at the Centre Claude Robillard and consisted of a choice of five events with total points the winner. I chose the 100 and 1500 metre races, the discus and javelin in the field event category and my favourite, the slalom.

I think I ended up 13th out of the 50 athletes, coming 5th in both the 100 and the 1500. The competition finished on a high note though as hometown athlete Doug Lyons topped the field of athletes.

When I came back from the competition in Quebec, I had to decide on my next plan of action, because it wasn't long after returning from Edmonton that I was let go from the Bell for taking too much time off. I couldn't afford the apartment any longer, but I was able to sublet the place to a couple of friends and they let me stay there until something came up.

Luckily, another basketball teammate offered me a place to stay for the winter, and so I moved to a small house just north of Fenelon Falls in October of '77. Saved my bacon no doubt but living up north meant the only training I got was when I travelled down into Toronto for ball practice or games, since a main highway passed in front of their house, and it was too dangerous to wheel on the road.

In what was supposed to be a great time for me after my record-breaking trip to Edmonton, it instead found me alone and depressed. The more I partied, the worse I felt. I had thought my life was beginning to settle down and good things were on the horizon, but they were either great or horrible and I was not sure which side was going to win out. No job, no place of my own, and alone. It was a bad trifecta.

Chapter 8:
Overcoming Obstacles

One day in early spring, while I was in Peterborough shopping, I ran across a friend who happened to know of an upstairs apartment in a small house for rent in town. It was cheap enough that I could afford it on my disability pension, and even though I had to leave my wheelchair at the bottom of the stairs, I couldn't stay in Fenelon Falls indefinitely. Being in town meant my ex was around somewhere, and for some reason, it made me feel better.

But the move to Peterborough presented the same challenge I had up in Fenelon Falls, no track to train on. I was unable to find an accessible track in the whole city, so I headed out on the road instead. Except for the hill climbing I did when I lived in Toronto, training on the road was a new experience for me. While American wheelers had been racing on the road even before Bob Hall's historic Boston Marathon wheel in '75, it had not caught on in Canada to any great extent.

With no job, I was free to wheel late at night when there was minimal traffic to contend with, and I got in the habit of leaving my apartment near George and Lansdowne Streets after dark and heading uptown. I wheeled up the main drag, turned right at the local Tim Hortons, crossed the bridge over the Otonabee River, and made a left onto Armor Road which soon turned into the River Road.

By then I was almost out of Peterborough and heading for Lakefield. I stayed on this road with the Otonabee River on my left and followed it past Trent University, and along the way I wheeled past the Kawartha locks at Nassau Mills, Otonabee, Duoro and Sawer Creek. I kept rolling along the River Road to the edge of Lakefield until I reached the liquor store parking

Chapter 8: Overcoming Obstacles

lot. Dad was manager of the store in those days, and it was a good spot to take a break.

Sometimes I would cruise up the deserted main street before turning around and other times I would just chill in the parking lot and have some refreshments there before heading back to my apartment. They were tough workouts because I took out all my frustration and mental pain as I wheeled my way down the road, but, somewhere, somehow, it became more therapeutic than actual training. I found myself wheeling for miles and miles with no real purpose. It usually took me a good two to three, sometimes four hours to complete my run. I felt confident heading into the provincials.

The Ontario Games in Windsor were successful in that I won my events, but my times were not comparable to Edmonton. Without hard competition at the provincial level, I wasn't worried about getting picked for the nationals in St. John's Newfoundland, but I knew I'd have to get my butt in gear if I planned on being competitive on the Rock.

However, living in the same town as my ex-girlfriend was more of a distraction than I had anticipated, and while I physically wheeled miles and miles in my chair, my mind was a million miles away. My endurance was great, but I took it easy without realizing it. Going for a Sunday drive as it were, regardless of its length, was not getting me in the kind of shape I needed to be in for a sprinter. And so, I flew to Newfoundland with the Ontario team, hoping for good results.

The results were mixed at best. I managed a bronze in the 100 and silver in my 200 – 400 – 800 and 1500 metre races. A slalom silver and a basketball bronze rounded out the haul.

Fortunately for me, it was enough to get me on the team to Rio de Janeiro as the second Class 4, behind Alberta's Ron Minor, who had cleaned up this time. But it took Graham's assurance that I'd be ready in November to make the team. I needed some serious work, but my mind was still focused elsewhere.

With no track to wheel on, I continued to follow my road course when I got back from the nationals but threw in some sprints as I wheeled down the road. I was fortunate that the weather held out and I had no snow to contend with.

About a month before the team was about to leave for Brazil, I made my usual right turn at the donut shop and began my climb up the hill. I was on the sidewalk at this point, not paying attention to where I was going, and I nearly ran her down.

My route had unknowingly passed by my ex's grandmother's house, and the lady had seen me numerous times as I wheeled past on the sidewalk. She had mentioned it to her granddaughter, who I guess, knew through another friend that I was living in town. She waited one night at her grandmother's, to see if I would pass by.

That night, I told her I was training for the Pan Am Games in Brazil. She said she missed me, and since we were both in her hometown now, perhaps things would work out better the second time around. Perhaps.

Once the snow began to fall, I had to rely on my weight-lifting workouts to keep me in shape and hoped it would be enough. I kept on training, but now I had a bit of a spring in my step as I got ready to go to Rio. Had Fate tipped in my favour for a change?

We flew out of Toronto but had to land in Miami to pick up some of the American athletes and that meant an extra hour stuck in our seats before we left again. With all our chairs stored in the underbelly, it would have been a nightmare if we would have had to transfer to another plane, but luckily, we didn't have to disembark as the Customs officers came on board to check our passports.

Other than the stop-over, the flight was rather routine. Some people played cards, most of the veterans tried to sleep the time away. The rookies? They had their faces pressed to the windows as best they could. 'Course as we got closer to Brazil, the fantastic view of the ocean and its turquoise water had everyone jockeying for position to take pictures. Of all the trips I would take in my career, flying to Rio was one of the longest, but boasted the most amazing scenery as we were arriving.

Clearing customs took no time at all and we were soon on the army buses, heading for our accommodations. A twenty-minute ride and we pulled up to the gates.

The first glimpse of our home away from home gave us more than a few reservations though. This was no one-star hotel. Seems we were going

Chapter 8: Overcoming Obstacles

to be housed in the old army barracks, the operative word being old. In Canada, they would have been condemned.

We were told that, prior to our arrival, the barracks had been emptied and given the once-over with flamethrowers to eliminate most of the bugs and the like. Then the inside was whitewashed. Ceiling, walls...everything white.

Each section had rows of metal bunk beds, with a slab of foam for a mattress, and a thin blanket. With the temperatures hovering in the mid 80's, if not higher at night, I hardly thought I would need a blanket. I was wrong.

Our building housed the men's Mexican team athletes, part of the American squad and us. While the Mexican team seemed unfazed by their surrounding, the Americans began to revolt. The accommodations were not acceptable, and they voiced their displeasure at the conditions.

We were not thrilled by any means, but in the beginning, we tried to make the best of it. Those of us who were mobile enough to climb, took to the top bunks.

Sitting up there, I couldn't help but notice that the dozens of windows that lined the upper half of the long side wall, did not have any glass in them. Are there mosquitos in Brazil? Does a bear poop in the woods?

As night fell for the first time, you could hear them outside, staging their assault. Squadrons upon squadrons of mosquitoes and who knows what else. What they were, mattered not, we were defenceless.

That first night was something I have never experienced again, and I've spent many a night under the stars during fishing season in the Kawarthas. Flying bugs came in through the windows and sucked the blood out of us all night long. We couldn't wait for daylight. When it did come, we realized bed bugs had chewed any of the leftover surfaces that the mosquitoes had missed. It was the last we saw of the American team. They were moved to a hotel.

So, everyone began the first day in Rio with little or no sleep, each one of us hoping it was not our event that was starting things off. We all filed onto the buses for the ride to the stadium where the competitions were scheduled to be held and where food was served and where the dreaded classification was to take place. Oh, and the slalom was the very first event.

Coming here, we knew beforehand that political unrest in Brazil had become a concern, to the point that there had been talk of cancellation, or of moving the Games somewhere else. There were fears by the Government that these games might be an opportunity, with North America watching, to abduct or harm an athlete as a means of having their agenda heard. The result of it all meant the stadium was closed to everyone except officials, team members and other accredited individuals. It was just us.

First up was classification. The Stoke Mandeville Federation had decided to revise the classification system once again, after the Toronto competition, and with the next set of Paralympics set for Holland in 1980, the national teams from all countries wanted to be sure their athletes were classified correctly to avoid challenges later.

Canada and United States had all their experienced doctors there in Rio, so everyone knew the classification we received at this competition, would be the class we would be in for the foreseeable future. Most athletes expected to stay in the same class, but there was a few of us that were borderline. Now that the system had been fine-tuned, if you will, it would all depend upon where we fit in the new points system, which was beginning to recognize the difference between the classes by how they performed their individual event, as well as their apparent impairment level.

When it was my turn, and the two American doctors had finished their assessment, I was stunned that both doctors agreed with what our doctors had determined; I was borderline Class 3/4 , and after a second examination, I had been dropped down to a Class 3. I would have no more medicals for the foreseeable future. Excellent. But competition would still be stiff.

My dropping down a class meant a change to the team structure as well, since now Ron and I were in different classes and would not be competing against each other. Hopefully, that meant a better chance of adding to the team's medal count.

It also meant a change in the events I could be entered in. At this competition, the lower classes were only allowed to wheel up to the 400 metres, which meant I lost out in wheeling the 1500. The 800 and the 1500 were going to be contested by the Class 4 - 5 racers. I had to be satisfied with wheeling the 100 and 400, plus the slalom and playing basketball.

Dropping down a class was an unexpected team bonus, but I realized I was still in over my head, when I went out on the track for the first time and began to warm up with the crew. Ron was in top shape and national team

Chapter 8: Overcoming Obstacles

rookie Mel Fitzgerald was destined to make history before we would leave South America, and between the two of them they led the team around the track at a good clip. But after only a few laps, I was struggling to keep up to the teams' pace. That was a bad sign.

Although I had ramped up my training when I got back from the nationals, road work, no matter how much you do, does not get you track-ready. Graham was not a happy camper. He was angry with me because he went to bat for me after my less than stellar showing in St. John's. Girl problems were not his problem.

He banished me from training with the guys and I was to work out when everyone was gone. That meant after all the teams had finished doing their workouts, I went on the track and tried to get as much training in as possible. The races were scheduled at the end of the games, so I had more than a few days to find my missing gear, if that was possible.

First gear was not there as evident when Graham and I did a bunch of starts that first day. My initial reaction time was slow and so was the time it took me to hit top speed. If I had been racing the 1500, I might have been better off, since a lightning-quick start would not be as critical. But, as it stood, I needed to get out of the gate quickly and push hard for just one lap.

Of course, the American track team had been there bright and early to watch and gauge the speed and depth of the other teams, especially our guys. And we looked impressive, well except for me. I must have stood out like a sore thumb because practise had just ended when a US racer with arms like a linebacker, rolled over to inform me of what he had planned to do to me during our races. "You can't even stay with your teammates warming up, I am going to..." And more words to that effect. My coach had just embarrassed me in front of the track team, but this guy made me angry. Angry that I had allowed my brain to get off track for so many months, angry that I had showed up in less than peak condition. Angry that I hadn't been able to find an accessible track to train on. But I had a slight window of opportunity to work with and work I did. I needed my jump, I needed it like yesterday.

But first things first, I had the slalom to wheel at the end of that first day and having won a bronze in Toronto in '76, I was hoping to improve on the color of the medal if I could. And the way things were going I thought it might well be the only chance for a medal this time around. It might be the only chance to save face.

It was obvious that the biggest challenge would come from American Dave Williamson. In warm-up he was moving around quite quickly and doing it in a chair set-up like I had never seen before. Instead of the regular 24" rear wheels we were used to seeing on slalom chairs, Dave was riding on 20" wheels, with a pair of small hand-rims. Was this déjà vu all over again? I got burned in Toronto with big wheels, were small wheels now going to be my downfall?

Unlike his teammate, Dave was a quiet confident athlete who found no reason to trash talk. He told me the smaller wheels lowered his centre of gravity and allowed him to slide around the pylons easier, without feeling like he might tip over from the momentum that builds up as you go through the course. Great idea. Why didn't I think of that!

As usual, before the race, we drew numbers to see what order we would compete in. I drew a high number and therefore got to watch most of the athletes perform before my turn came up.

Dave wheeled a smooth no-penalty run and looked like a lock for the gold, but I had other ideas when it was my turn. I touched nothing as well, and I knew it was a fast time, but it wasn't until I crossed the finish line that I realized I had made a serious blunder. I had gone the wrong way around the very last pylon on the way to the finish line. I was disqualified. No medal of any colour.

While Ron and Joanne MacDonald came back to the barracks with gold medals from their slalom event, I had nothing to show for my effort. That night was the low point of my career. I began to think I should have stayed home. Sitting up there in my top bunk, listening to the guys recount their results from the day, I could hardly mutter my apologies for my blunder. I only hoped that the mosquitoes drowned out the sound of my tears of frustration.

While the American team left the barracks as soon as possible, we carried on as best we could. But after the third or fourth night, I can't remember which, word came that we were moving to a hotel just off Ipanema Beach.

Talk about one extreme to another. The hotel was great. Swimmer/basketball player Laurie Hersom from St Catherine's was my roommate.

Chapter 8: Overcoming Obstacles

We had played ball against each other and as teammates on the provincial squad on numerous occasions, and we got along well. Lucky for me, I had quit swimming by now, and was not required to race in the pool of murky green coloured water that he was scheduled to compete in.

We were fortunate that our hotel room had a balcony that you could go out on for fresh air if it got too stuffy. With the lobby below us to the right, there was another room on the other side, with its own balcony, and on the first day we arrived, there was a beautiful girl out there sunbathing. She could only speak Spanish but showing her my uniform, she knew I was from Canada.

Her name was Guadalupe and we tried to have conversations every day. I figured she was eighteen if that, but regardless of our age difference, we had fun trying to converse with each other nonetheless.

Being so close to the beach was great as well. Ipanema Beach is one of the most famous beaches in the world and the 2km long boardwalk made of smooth stones was great to wheel along.

The beach stretches 2 km between Jardim de Alah and Arpoador, where a giant stone separates it from Copacabana Beach. Both the boardwalks were created by Brazilian architect Roberto Bublé Marx in 1971, and his design on both boardwalks, was his abstract interpretation of a traditional Portuguese paving pattern, using black and white stones. Its breathtaking to sit at one end near the giant rock and look down on the boardwalk as it stretches back towards Jardim de Alah.

During one wheel, Ron Minor and I decided to travel the whole length of the boardwalk. Dressed in our Canadian singlets, with a bit of coconut oil to "keep us from burning", we headed out.

One thing we quickly noticed as we wheeled along was the various metal workout stations that were set up in the sand along the edge of the boardwalk. As people strolled past, big muscular guys would do chin-ups and hanging crunches to the appreciation of the thong-clad ladies that stood around watching.

We stopped at one of the stations and watched as a couple of guys did chin-ups. I looked at Ron and said "What do you think? Show 'em how Canadians do them?"

Ron was always up for some fun, so we left our chairs on the boardwalk and crawled across the sand, pulled ourselves up the metal side poles and moved into the centre. Hanging side by side, we pulled off a dozen or so one-handed chin-ups, dropped to the sand and made our way back into our chairs.

Claps and big smiles from the gals were part of our reward, as was knowing none of the guys were going to attempt any more feats of strength... until we rolled on.

But back to the task at hand. Not for one minute had I forgotten the situation I had put myself in. I wheeled as much as possible, consisting of short bursts of sprinting and working on my initial take-off. I knew I'd have to get off the line as fast as I could if I wanted a chance at a medal. These races were not going to be a two-country showdown, by any means. The Mexican and Brazilian teams would have a say in the matter, and there was always a lot of competitors from all countries in the sprints.

I always thought, rightly or wrongly, that my being only 90 pounds was an advantage in that I felt like I could get in shape faster than those who had a much larger body mass. Would I see results? Not sure. But I wheeled alone. I barfed alone. And I told myself while I was alone and race day was finally upon us, that some measure of success was not out of the realm of possibility, because I did feel that my acceleration had been turned up a notch. I was beginning to peak, and I was lucky as it turned out.

Everyone who knows me, knows I am a junk food junkie. I'll take a large bag of chips and a chocolate bar over steak and potatoes any day. And being born disabled, I knew my body well, just out of necessity. Like what food I could eat without having an unfavourable reaction later. Changes in food effect people in different ways but being disabled it often meant that it didn't take much to upset the system. So, it wasn't much of a surprise when athletes began to have stomach disorders of the # 2 kind.

I think it was the third day that I sat down at lunch with part of the team, since I was usually off wheeling somewhere, fueled by my stash of jellybeans, ju jubes, chocolate bars and the rest of the junk food I brought with me. But Graham had come over to me earlier in the day to tell me he had only banished me from training with the guys and not to let that spoil the rest of the experience.

Chapter 8: Overcoming Obstacles

On this day lunch consisted of a bowl of rice with chunks of meat and black peas of some sort. I said that the meat looked a tad green in spots, don't you think? But being hungry at that moment, and enjoying sitting with the team for a change, I thought what the heck.

What followed was probably one of the funniest things I've ever experienced on a games trip. Before I had taken a bite of the meat, I said out loud, "Why do the black peas have tiny legs?" The look on everyone's face at the table when they uncurled a "pea", only to expose little beetle legs, was priceless.

Unfortunately, and not the least bit funny, was the fact that the bad food ruined a lot of performances by many athletes while we were there. Some of my teammates returned home empty-handed because they had no strength left to compete successfully. Just one variable that the disabled had to contend with when competing out-of-country. Junk food saved me, this time .

Finally, race day arrived. It was hotter than a firecracker and not a lick of wind nor a cloud in the sky. Track was old but it was nice and hard and by the look of the wheelers that I watched train I thought that records might be set before the games were over. If we could overcome the temperature that continued to climb as the day went on.

First up for me was the 400, and Graham had told me that our heat would be the quickest, so he wanted me to go all out to ensure it would be enough to make the final. I don't think he had watched me train and I don't think he was convinced that I could go all out, twice in a row, with the same result, but he wanted to ensure I made the final at least.

I didn't get the best start and that resulted in coming fourth, but with the American athlete leading the way, it was the quickest of all the heats and good enough to get me in the final.

As luck would have it, I drew lane one for the final. I like lane one. The US was out in lane 4 and I had a good view of the whole field to start the race. A fast Brazilian athlete was in one of the lanes between us. I knew from watching the American during his training sessions that, like my teammate Ron Minor, he was more brute strength than technique, and while he could surely motor down the straights, his speed into the corners forced him to bounce his front end up and around to stay in his lane and that slowed him down somewhat.

It was my hope that with a full head of steam going down the backstretch, the utilization of my one-hand steering technique would take me around the tight lane one corner as smoothly as possible, and hopefully set me up at the head of the stretch for a mad dash for a medal.

Before the race I went over strategy with Graham. He said I had to put pressure on the American right away, or he would breeze to victory. I had to get close enough to him to force him to react to my presence. Then anything can happen.

I knew what he really meant though. Try and chase this guy down and perhaps it will get me past the rest of the pack and into the medals. Better than nothing…like the slalom.

The gun sounded and off we went. As predicted, the US surged into the lead with Brazil not far behind. Halfway down the back stretch I overtook the athlete from South America and found myself a couple of chair lengths behind the US. By the time we reached the corner I had cut the lead to a chair length and rolling in lane one, I flew around the final corner. Steering with my left hand and using maybe 7-8 strokes, I came out of the corner as smooth as silk. More importantly, I had gained ground.

Hopping the front end of his chair to get around the corner had indeed cost my American opponent a little off his top end speed, and with about a chair length to make up as I came out of the corner, I picked up the pace as he bolted for home. Half-way down the straightaway I was closing in on his back wheels.

This was the pivotal point of the race. Did I have enough to sustain the push? In Lane 1, I was out of my competitor's view as he was only focused on the finish line. With about 10 to 15 chair lengths from the tape, I turned up my push rate to max and fanned my rims as fast as I possibly could. I'm not sure if he ran out of gas, let up because he thought he had it in the bag, or my last surge with a couple of metres to go, caught him by surprise. Regardless, I closed the gap and won by the length of a footplate.

Coasting around the corner with my index finger raised high, Graham stood on the sidelines with a stunned look on his face, while my competitor was, at best, none too pleased. "Should have been a Class 4" was his first

Chapter 8: Overcoming Obstacles

reaction. "Sandbagging" was what he said to me later. I faked being slow to throw him off.

Not really. Maybe I just wanted it more, needed it more. I felt pressure to make up for my slalom blunder that cost us a medal in the team standings. However, he made it perfectly clear that regardless of this outcome, the 100 would be a different story.

The 100 is one of the most anticipated races and with it brings bragging rights. Winning the 100 means you're the fastest in the world for that sliver of time. Being the 100 metre champion is a special honour.

Frankly, I didn't much care at that moment. The pressure was off my shoulders, and I felt like I had redeemed myself somewhat. Anything else was gravy. Always lots of athletes that were quick in the 100 and it is a race that's usually very unforgiving. The 100 is a scary race and naturally the most fun! I'd take what I could get.

But for now, I was basking in the fun of winning. I can still picture the giant scoreboard flashing in the centre of the infield...CHRIS... CANADA...1:21.0...PAN AM RECORD. Yee haw!! My winning time was not close to my personal best but under the oppressive heat and melting track, it was good enough. And more than anyone expected.

In late afternoon, with the temperature reaching triple digits, it was time for the 100 metres. You could see the heat waves coming off the softened track as we prepared to race. As expected, there were a lot of heats to get through before the real action started, and though you just want to go fast enough to make the finals, it's a fine line. Save too much and you may find that too many athletes went wide open, and you didn't even make the semi-final. Go too fast and your final might be slower, depending upon your fitness level.

Besides the oppressive heat, there was a problem with the consistency of the starter. He wasn't. Sometimes he'd say "ON YOUR MARK, GET SET"...and then the gun would go off. Other times it was "ON YOUR MARK" and then boom, you'd be left at the line. The coaches tried to no avail to get it consistent, but it remained hit or miss.

My American competitor was in my heat again, and we got the quick start, which he anticipated. He vanished in an instant. "Holy Crap" I thought to myself. Talk about putting it in gear. It was a mad push as I wheeled down that straightaway. He had a big lead, and coming out of the gate dead last, I realized I had 6 others to reel in or there might not be a final for me. I finished 4th but lucky for me, our heat was by far the quickest again, so I made the final 8.

When it was our turn for the final, I drew lane 2 with the US occupying lane 4. Although hoping the starter would get it right, I was prepared for a quick start, but when it happened, I still hesitated slightly, and I was instantly behind. US took the lead.

A quarter of the way down the straight I found myself in 4th or 5th and by the halfway point, I had passed all but one. I was still a good chair-length back though and running out of real estate.

I began to close the gap and again, I don't think he heard me until he saw me out of the corner of his eye, because the US team had stationed themselves just past the finish line on the right side and they were cheering like mad. He tried to pick up the pace when he felt my presence, but it was too late. The margin of victory was all of 3 inches this time.

My heartbeat had still not gone down to normal when that scoreboard flashed once more...CHRIS...CANADA...21 sec...PAN AM RECORD. Again, not the fastest I had wheeled the 100, but it was enough. Sometimes, it's not the time it takes, but who gets to the line first.

What caught my attention was the fact that the times for both my finals had the number 21 in them. Twenty-one had been my basketball number since I began playing with the Thunderbolts and 21 had been worn by my favorite baseball player, the great Roberto Clemente. It was also the day of my girlfriend's birthday. Were the stars aligning in my favour?

Of course, the two gold that I managed to win paled in comparison to the rest of what the track team accomplished. Ron cleaned up in Class 4 with multiple gold in his individual events and silver in the relay to take home to Alberta, and in what was the most thrilling race of the games, Mel Fitzgerald earned his "Newfie Bullet" moniker when he became the first wheelie to post a sub-5-minute 1500 metre, winning the Class 5 event in 4:59.3. Sweet. I told people it could be done. Glad it was a fellow Canadian and a great guy that proved me right.

While results from this competition were difficult to come by, on the women's side, besides her slalom gold, I know Joanne won a silver in the

60 and the 1500 metres, with a bronze thrown in for a 3rd place finish in the 800.

Joanne also went back to Newfoundland with a medal that none of the guys who played basketball could stake claim to, as the Canadian women's basketball team won silver in the final against a strong US squad.

Both the men and women's teams had to settle for silver in the relays, but it was a successful outing overall. Most everyone went home happy with the results.

Rio was the only time I played on the National basketball team and my best memory of the round-robin was dropping 20 points vs Venezuela in one of our victories. Unfortunately, we were shut out of the medals this time around, but I thought we played well considering the team had been thrown together on short notice. But the Canadian team, both men and women would win gold in the coming years as our basketball program kicked into high gear.

Regardless of where I travelled with the team, I always managed to have some sort of adventure before we headed for home. My first instance came before we moved out of the barracks to the hotel near Ipanema Beach.

A few of us wanted to go for a wheel and see the sights late one afternoon. The armed guard at the gate gave us some stern advice before we headed out though. The most important being that we got back before it got dark. If we were out there in the dark, there was more than a good chance of us vanishing, never to be seen again. And we were not to go far into the little village that was at the end of the road that we were going to wheel on. That would be dangerous as well. Our clothes would be enough to draw attention that we were tourists, and off the beaten track, no-one was safe. He seemed a bit paranoid to me, but what did I know?

We took his words to heart and headed down the road. For about an hour, we wheeled along, taking in everything we could see. We were enjoying ourselves so much that we didn't realize how much time had passed and it was getting dark. Starting to get a little paranoid ourselves, we began to head back to the barracks.

The sun went down quickly, fast enough that we found ourselves still on the road at dusk, and it didn't take long for us to start to become apprehensive. All along the road, there was garbage everywhere, in bags, or just thrown on the ground in piles. And now there seemed to be movement among these piles of refuse. Soon, we began to see little eyes in the fading light, staring at us as we went past, and it wasn't long before some of the eyes began to follow us from shadow to shadow as we wheeled down the road.

Then suddenly the guard from the barracks appeared out of the darkness, and he was none too pleased with us. He said we knew better than to stray too far since the country's political unrest might make us targets and we should have gotten back sooner.

He also said the sounds we heard and the eyes we saw coming from the garbage were either wild dogs that roamed the streets or the massive rats that lived in the junk. He said that eventually they would have attacked us.

I thought that was a bit of a stretch, but the look on his face gave me pause for thought and it gave me a chill down my spine all the same. If he hadn't gone looking for us, I shudder to think what our Fate might have been. Getting bitten by something would not have been good.

One day the same guard asked me if I would trade my Canada hat for one of his pistols and its holster. I was never into guns but thought it would be a cool souvenir. Luckily, I asked one of my coaches and he said we had to keep our gear until the games were over, not to mention handguns were illegal in Canada and I could get in all kinds of trouble if I tried to get it over the border. Good thing I asked. But once the games were finished, I found him and gave him my hat. No big deal, but I was grateful that he thought enough to go looking for us.

There were no more unauthorized side trips anywhere, but I still manage to get in hot water when all I wanted to do was see a soccer game.

Some of us were offered tickets to see a game between a team from Brazil and their arch-rivals from Argentina. I didn't follow soccer, but I had heard about the famous Maracanã Stadium, and I didn't want to miss the chance to see a game there.

The stadium was opened the day I was born, June 16th 1950, as a result of Brazil being award the FIFA World Cup. The stadium was constructed with a wide 20-foot ditch or moat that separated the playing field from the stands. While spectators filled the stadium through the turnstiles, the players emerged from a tunnel leading up to the field. No chance for people to storm the field for whatever reason. With a seating capacity estimated to be over 200,000 people, it was the largest stadium in the world at the time.

Outside the stadium, they were selling cushions of both teams. The stadium is solid concrete, and the cushions supplied some comfort for your butt. I didn't have a favourite team, but I liked the blue and white striped cushions, so Laurie and I each bought one and headed inside.

Not long after the game had started, we noticed people around us were starting to give us a hard time. They began yelling at us and throwing stuff in our direction. Things were starting to get ugly, and my wheelchair had been moved to another area, so I was stuck where we were. Just when we were starting to get nervous, a man came down from the stands to talk to us. Did we know that we were sitting in the Brazilian section, waving Argentinian cushions around? No wonder the fans were ticked off!

Well, I knew what to do once I realized what was going on. We held up our cushions for the fans to see, spit on them, and threw them into the moat surround the playing field. Our section erupted in cheers and two gentlemen came down and gave us their cushions to sit on. Whew, crisis averted. Good thing we had our Canadian jackets on!

On the day we were to leave, the bus pulled up and we climbed aboard in preparation for the ride to the airport. Our chairs were stored underneath the bus, as usual, and I was just getting comfortable, when one of our coaches came on board and said someone was looking for me. I looked out the window of the bus, and there was Guadalupe, with a present in hand.

My chair was packed away so I opened the window, and hung out as far as I could, but I was still too high. Ron to the rescue. While holding my ankles, he lowered me down the side of the bus until I was low enough for her to kiss me on the cheek and put something in my hand.

It was totally unexpected, and I was at a loss for words, but I remembered the pendant and chain I bought while out shopping.

Rio's good luck charm seemed to be a closed fist with the index finger extended, as if you were saying I'm #1. I had bought myself a gold one and a chain to go with it as a souvenir. I undid the clasp and dropped it into her hand, and Ron pulled me back into the bus amid a chorus of good-natured ribbing. Once back in my seat, I opened my present to find a 45-record, "The Girl from Ipanema." Enclosed was a picture and her address.

We wrote back and forth for awhile, but somewhere along the line I lost the address and never heard from her again. I still have the "45" though.

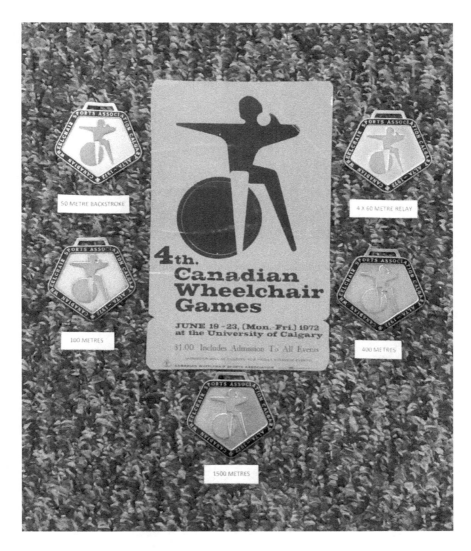

72 Calgary Nationals Program

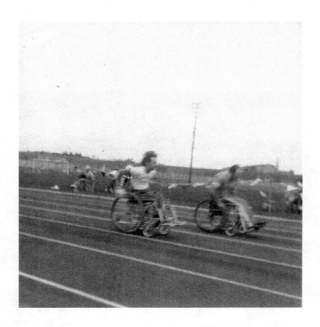

Overtaking Rene Massé of Quebec for the silver medal in the 100-metre final at the '72 Calgary Nationals

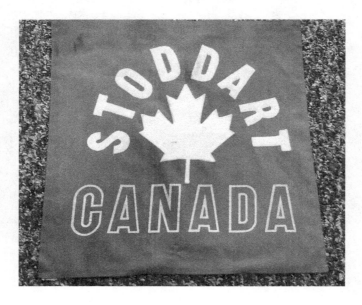

My Paralympic chairback

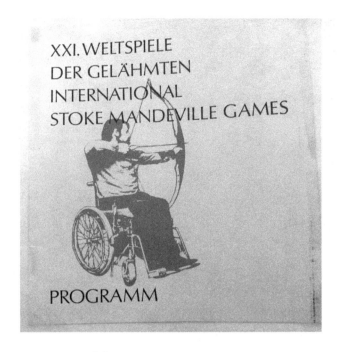

Heidelberg Germany Games program

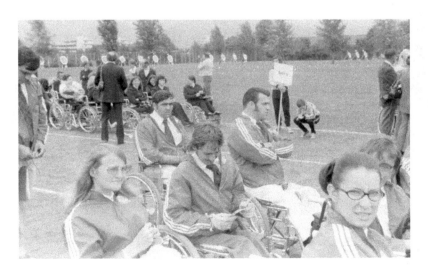

Lining up for opening ceremonies in Heidelberg (l-r) Sandy Davenport - Reg Muise - Chris Stoddart - Gene Reimer - Hilda Binns - Joyce Murland

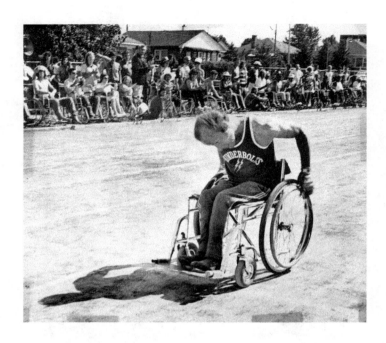

Canada's 1st 100 metre Paralympic champion - Bob Simpson

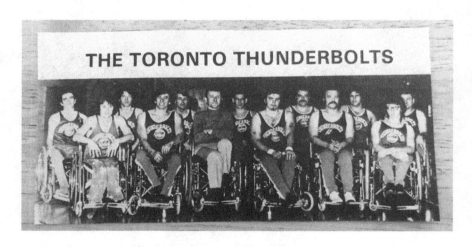

Toronto Thunderbolts team roster (l-r) (back row) Dunc Wilson – John Crawford – Bob Lowe – Peter Hand – Gord Paterson – Bill Brouse – Dave Jack (front row) Chris Stoddart – Eddie Litzenberger – Bev Hallam – Brian Halliday – Dale Moe – Mike O'Brien

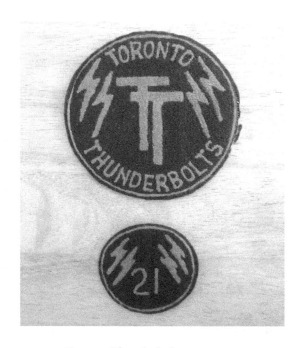

Toronto Thunderbolts team crest

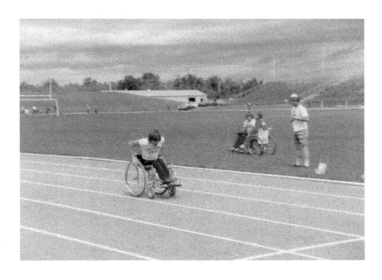

Pushing to victory in the class 4 400 metre final at the 74 Winnipeg National Games

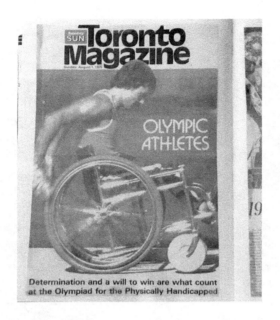

Toronto Sun cover promoting the 1976 TorontOlympiad

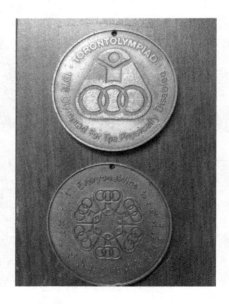

My bronze medals from the 800 metre and the slalom competition at the 1976 Paralympics

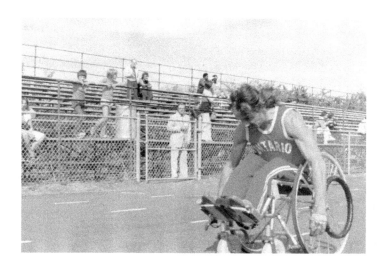

Heading for gold in my new racer during the 1500 metre final at the 1977 Edmonton National Games

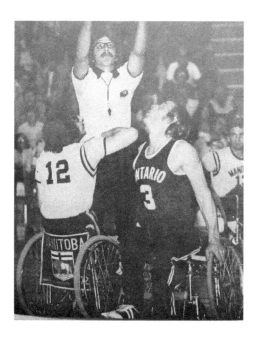

Manitoba's John Lundie and Ontario's Flo Aukema prepare for the tipoff of the 1977 Canadian Wheelchair Basketball Championships, won by Ontario

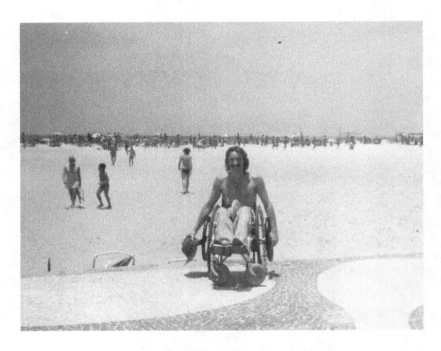

Relaxing on Ipanema beach after winning gold in the 100 and 400 metre at the 1978 Rio de Janeiro Pan American Wheelchair Games

Chapter 9:
Calm Before the Storm

Back home after returning from Rio, it wasn't long before the "ex" became the "ex-ex" and she moved in with me once more. Life was good again.

It was a great winter, and in the spring, she told me of a provincial program aimed at getting families into houses that they could rent-to-own. She thought we might qualify, even though I was living off my disability pension and she was on unemployment insurance. Seemed a longshot but the CMHC representative took us for a ride out into the country to see the place and before I knew it, we were moving in.

Since I was going to be away at competitions throughout the year, she wanted us to get a dog for protection for when I was away. A friend of hers in town had Doberman pincher puppies for free, so I said to pick the biggest one. Soon after, we came home with a big chubby pup curled up inside my leather jacket.

As was the custom back then, we had his ears cropped and his tail shortened, and being a huge Star Trek fan, I called him Mr. Spock. Anyone that knew me back then, will remember him fondly. He was a great dog and loved virtually everybody.

Moving into a house instead of living in a second-floor apartment was great. We had a big back yard, but the row of houses was new enough that there was no fencing behind us or between any of the places along the street. My first trick was teaching Mr. Spock to poop on our property, since I got an earful when he dropped "his business" on a neighbour's lawn the first chance he had.

Life was good, but again, I was stuck in a place with nowhere to train. Workouts consisted of wheeling back and forth along the strip of uneven road that passed in front of the house. It was too dangerous wheeling on the main road because the sightlines were compromised by trees, and vehicles came up on me too quickly to allow for any time to get out of the way if need be.

So, I entered the '79 mid-June Oshawa Ontario Games in not the best of shape but good enough to sweep my events. Dropping down a class meant I was now racing athletes I had never competed against before, and that took some getting used to.

When I eventually flew to Richmond BC for the re-named Eleventh National Wheelchair Games, later in the year, I was introduced to two future members of our Canadian track team, Class 4 racers Andre Viger from Quebec, and an athlete from Williams Lake BC, by the name of Rick Hansen.

For some reason, my new classification was not recognized at the Nationals that year, but regardless, five bronze were all I managed to cart home from out West. That didn't surprise me really, considering everything I had been going through, but I was ticked off considerably when I crashed and burned my way through a penalty-filled run in my favourite event, the slalom. There was no excuse for that.

While my Class 3 designation was finally recognized by the end of the year, Andre had also been reclassified down to Class 3 and my poor showing in Richmond left me as the third choice in my class, in line to make the '80 Holland Paralympic team. I couldn't help but think that perhaps the circumstances from Rio would dictate that I'd have to prove I had a chance to win a medal before I would be considered for a berth on any future team.

Back at the ranch, my girlfriend and I had a great first Christmas together in the new house. A bunch of teammates and friends came up from the city to party on New Year's Eve. The winter of '79 was rough in our neck of the woods, and it made for many a white-knuckle trip back into Toronto to play basketball, so I was more than ready when spring arrived.

Chapter 10:
House of Cards

April 12th 1980 was a special day in Canada as Terry Fox dipped his artificial leg into the Atlantic Ocean in St. John's NFLD for the first time and began his Marathon of Hope.

When he lost his leg at 18 to bone cancer, Terry decided that he wanted to raise money and awareness for cancer research. After training for nearly a year and a half with his friend Rick Hansen and playing on the Vancouver Cable Cars wheelchair basketball team, he set off across Canada as a beacon of hope. Hoping his efforts would raise enough money to help in the battle against the insidious disease. While there was limited press in the beginning, by the time he reached Thunder Bay on Sept 1st and had 143 days and almost 3,400 km under him, he was becoming a National hero to the millions of people touched by cancer.

I was getting ready to head into the city to play in the First Spitfire Challenge Basketball Tournament, when my girlfriend asked me if I thought my parents would take Mr. Spock for the days I was gone. She wanted to stay at her mom's place for the weekend and was worried that Mr. Spock might hurt her mom's little doggie.

Now Mr. Spock was as mellow a Doberman as you could find and at 8 months old, I had never seen him aggressive to anyone. But strangely, I had noticed that lately, he seemed to watch her as she walked around the house. Nonetheless, Mom and Dad had a way with dogs, and he never caused a problem when they babysat him for me.

Much later I found out that, I guess Mr. Spock had eaten a pair of slippers when I was gone one day, and she had picked him up and tossed him against the wall. That's why he kept on eye on her.

The Challenge was a wheelchair basketball tournament that the Spitfires created both to raise funds for their club, and to expose the value of having a fully integrated wheelchair basketball team. They advertised the fact that they had non-disabled players but with the thought that they would not impact the game to any great extent, numerous American NWBA teams would come north for the tournament.

Over the previous few years, the SOWBL had grown to include more teams in the league, and as I mentioned earlier, the league initially voted to allow able-bodied athletes to play wheelchair basketball because some new teams didn't have enough disabled players. It was assumed that the able-bodied players would be replaced by a disabled player when the opportunity presented itself, and since they were not very good in a wheelchair, they initially did nothing to alter the outcome of the games.

Funny thing though. Over time, they got much better and started to dominate. Their love of the game meant they put in as much, if not more time getting better. Especially the Spitfire players, who put forth the notion that there was nothing wrong with having able-bodied players on the team regardless of how many players were available.

The Spitfires were led by able-bodied players Bob Bryce and Jerry Tonello, both who spent countless hours playing wheelchair basketball. In the future, each one would earn the opportunity to coach our national teams to great success.

Since the NWBA did not allow able-bodied players, the US teams were none too happy when they realized just how good Bob and Jerry were. Combined with eventual national team member, Flo Aukema, the Spitfires were a near unbeatable team.

However, as years past, dozens of American teams would still travel across the border, often with All-Star teams to challenge the Spitfires. Eventually the Spitfire Challenge became one of the best wheelchair basketball tournaments ever.

Chapter 10: House of Cards

It was a 3-day basketball tournament but as well as basketball, there was a free-throw contest, spaghetti-eating contest, video game contests, all kinds of activities to make sure your trip to Toronto and the Spitfire Challenge was a memorable one. Usually, more than a half dozen teams made their way north of the border, to compete against the Spitfires and other teams based throughout Ontario and beyond. It was always a great tournament regardless of your team's success.

It was dark when I eventually got home and rolled into the driveway, and it was strange that there were no outside lights on. I thought maybe my girlfriend was still in town until I unlocked the front door and found the place half empty. Most of the furniture was gone including my stereo. At first, I thought we had been robbed, but as I went about the house, I realized only my clothes were left hanging in the closets.

I slept on the floor that night and told my parents the news when I went to pick up Mr. Spock the next morning. I went back a few days later and the locks had been changed. With no other recourse I went to the authorities and when I explained the situation and who the family was, they said I should consider myself lucky I only lost furniture. Turn the page and move on. So, I tried. But it wasn't easy. I moved back into my parent's place in Buckhorn while I figured out my next course of action.

I was devastated to say the least. As the days past I sunk lower and lower. Self destruction was the path I was heading down. I looked at my medal collection, wondering if I would win any more. I was brutally honest with myself. There was no motivation to be had. I lived at home with my parents at 29 years old, having screwed up two nice jobs with the Bell and now living on disability benefits.

The next few weeks were hell. The hardest part was being cheerful around my parents and pretending it was no big deal. Better now than later I'd say to anyone who asked. But I wondered if, or when, I would find someone who would love me forever instead of just for awhile. In the meantime, my racing chair gathered dust.

Then one day, I ran into old buddy Marv Murray. He had left his apartment in Don Mills where the group of us had lived, not long after I moved to Fenelon Falls and at that moment, he was sharing a townhouse in Scarborough with a couple of his buddies. They offered me and Mr. Spock a place to stay until I figured out what to do. What I wanted to do was crawl in a hole and disappear, but we moved in gratefully.

Wheelchair road racing in Ontario didn't begin until 1980, and the Oshawa Classic 10K was the first event that featured only disabled racers. Leaving from the Oshawa Civic Centre track, this first race had a half dozen or so wheelers lined up at the start line, though attendance grew every year. It usually ran in May and for athletes in Southern Ontario it marked a new beginning to the start of racing season.

I finished in 4th with a slow time after I was badgered by my buddies to get a grip and move on. How long was I going to sulk? So, I started wheeling again.

I did enjoy racing on the road though. It was a blast. Roads blocked off, cops directing traffic, people cheering as you raced past, what's not to like? Back then, actual wheelchair racing events were limited to say the least.

In Canada, we had provincials, nationals, and if you were good, Stoke Mandeville for the World Championships, or the Paralympics every four years. That was it. Then you waited for basketball season if that's how you passed the winter.

Meanwhile in America, road racing had become a big deal, with lots of races at all distances. And they competed in all kinds of racing chairs, often built by fellow racers. The summer in the southern States was endless. It was a wheelers paradise.

In the early years, with not many international competitions in a single season, most countries kept their secrets to themselves, and new techniques or equipment upgrades were not revealed until it was time to compete. Many countries were years behind, including Canada. Not until the early 80's when wheelchair marathon racing became more global, did the new ideas begin to reach more and more athletes.

Besides the disadvantages that the lack of sharing ideas on chair design, training and road racing technique that we didn't have up north caused, we missed out on the camaraderie that developed during road racing events. Meeting new friends in road races came years later.

In early July, in a second change of fortune, I got a job working for a company called Rainbow Gas in Mississauga. The company was owned

Chapter 10: House of Cards

by two brothers, and one brother had married one of the daughters of my dad's best friend from the War. They were up at the cottage visiting my parent's when I came up for the weekend and when Amadeo found out I was looking for work, he offered me a job and said I could bring Mr. Spock to work to act as the bodyguard for the unit where they built industrial heating and cooling systems. Excellent.

It came as no surprise when the call came advising me that I had not made the team going to Holland. With Andre reclassified down to a Class 3 and having only third place finishes from the Nationals in Richmond, the team decided to give someone else the opportunity.

It was a blow to my ego but should have been expected. I was given the benefit of the doubt once but not this time. The only meaningful competition on the track for me would be the Sault Ste. Marie Ontario Games, later in August.

Leading up to Holland my replacement had not expected to be picked and was not in shape for this calibre of competition. He had wheeled even less than me, but of course he didn't want to miss an opportunity to be a Paralympian.

Unfortunately, he started off on the wrong foot by missing the team plane going to Holland, and upon arriving a couple of days later, they realized that his racing chair needed work and would require more than a few hours with his trusty pop rivet gun to get it ready.

And while the chair held together, of course his fitness level was not comparable to the rest of the racers. With the likes of Rick Hansen, Mel Fitzgerald, Andre Viger, Paul Clark and Ron Minor in the mix, the air about the team was all business and the obvious lack of training and his habit of smoking cigarettes did not sit well with the guys.

At some point, I was contacted by Team Canada boss, the late great Barb Montemurro, and asked if I would be available to fly to Holland if a spot became available. I said yes. I wasn't near in top shape, but I knew I was the faster of the two of us, and I had years of international experience to rely on. I felt comfortable in agreeing to go if the opportunity presented itself.

While my new boss said no problem, Barb called a day later and said that Stoke rules stated that an athlete could only be substituted to replace another injured athlete in his class. Since the athlete was not injured, he could not be replaced, and so my slim chance to be part of the team that rolled onto the track in Holland was dashed for good.

Since the development of track was still ongoing, some athletes were again restricted on the distance they could compete in internationally, and Holland was no different. The quad racers were restricted more than the paras by a great deal. Back in America and in countries around the world, not only were quadriplegics racing all the track distances, but many had already taken to the roads, wheeling distances from the 10k to the full marathon. In Holland they were restricted to the 60-metre sprint only. It was just one example where a governing body hindered the development of wheelchair racing by taking so long to change their views.

In addition, while all the other classes raced the 100, only Class 2 and Class 3 athletes competed for the 200 and 400 titles and were denied the opportunity to race the 800 and 1500. Those were reserved for Classes 4-5 once more.

For the first time in international competition, there were no American quads that made the podium, as Mexico garnered 4 of the 9 available medals. Gary Birch was the lone Canadian medal winner, taking home the 60 metre Class 1A silver.

Marc de Myer of Belgium edged Canada's Mel Fitzgerald (18.07 vs 18.24) for gold in the Class 5 100 final. Erich Huber of Australia took home the bronze.

Canadian Class 4 Rick Hansen defeated veteran Brad Parks of the USA in the 800, winning in 2:25.92 for a world record. Uriel Martinez of Mexico won the bronze.

The 1500 final saw Parks returning the favour, edging out Rick for gold in 4:44.6. Belgian Remi van Ophen took home the bronze.

Mel Fitzgerald of Canada was golden in the 800 winning in 2:16.87 over Erich Hubel of Australia and Ebo Roek of The Netherlands, and he took another gold in the 1500 final over Roek and Hubel. While both Fitzgerald and Roek destroyed the existing record by wheeling under 5 minutes, Mel's time of 4:17:0 was a dominating win and served notice that the gold he won in Rio de Janeiro was just the beginning.

Chapter 10: House of Cards

Rick, Ron, Mel and Andre Viger combined to win bronze in the 4 x 100 metre relay, while Ron also won a bronze in the Class 4 slalom as did Ed Batt in Class 1C.

I took a mental note that Paul van Winkle of Belgium won the Class 3 slalom gold with Gregor Golombek of West Germany taking silver and Fred Pointer of Australia the bronze.

On the women's side, Joanne MacDonald won the Class 5 slalom title and Pam Frazee took home bronze in the Class 3 400 metre final.

Coming back from Holland, the guys had some great ideas for building the next generation racing chair. Rule changes from Holland finally gave us a little more leeway in building racers, and by the time the next Paralympics rolled around in '84, athletes from around the world would be competing in new state-of-the-art machines.

So, after we had competed in the Sault Ste. Marie Nationals, Billy and I decided to pool our resources with another athlete and together with our basketball teammate, Doug, the 3 of us would come up with three great chairs in time for next year's nationals that were scheduled for Scarborough.

Near the end of summer, the lease on the townhouse in Scarborough where we all lived was about to expire and all the guys were moving out at the end of September. I was going to have to find another place to live that would take Mr. Spock. As it turned out, he was not used to being by himself, and after eating the living room couch while I left him alone to go training one day, I moved out early and the two of us began to live in my car.

I changed my clothes and showered at the Etobicoke Olympium in Mississauga where the Spitfire Challenge was held, and at night I found a place to park the car that was safe but out of the way. In the two months or so that I slept in my car, I was only woken up by the police once. I explained to the officer that I worked in the city but lived in Buckhorn and was too tired to drive home that night. When Mr. Spock came out of the sleeping bag when he first knocked on the window, it convinced him I was in no danger and off he went.

I lived in my car with Mr. Spock until an article about my situation was printed in one of the newspapers and I was offered an apartment that would take the both of us. I gratefully moved into a rent-regulated apartment in the David B. Archer Co-op on the Esplanade near the St. Lawrence Market in December of '80. Downtown Toronto was a great place and I lived there for more than a decade.

Wheelchair basketball in Canada took another major step forward in '80 when Ontario was awarded its own Division in the NWBA to start the 80/81 basketball season. Kitchener Twin-City Spinners, London Forest City Flyers, Niagara Bullets, and the new Scarborough Hawks, competed in the newly created Lake Ontario Conference. As ball players, we were pumped to start a new chapter in wheelchair basketball and looked forward to not having to make the drive into the US unless we got in the playoffs.

The Hawks, who were basically the SOWBL Falcons with better uniforms, were headed by veteran Dale Moe and the rest of the players in the Toronto area that weren't members of the Spitfires. Our team gained a couple and lost a couple of players to start the season but were still looking for good results. Since the Spitfires were intent on making able-bodied players a permanent fixture in wheelchair basketball, they declined to join the first year.

As well we had two new volunteers to start the season. Jacquie Phillips and Bev Waddell were both high school students that were about to graduate. Bev was volunteering at the Scarborough Rec Club for Disabled Adults where teammate Dale Moe worked. He invited them to help with the Hawks.

The new NWBA season began during the Oktoberfest Festival Tournament in Kitchener in October, and games during this round-robin tournament counted in the league standings. Billy's mom's place in Kilbride was close enough to Kitchener, and with his mom being away for the weekend, he invited the team to stay there during the tournament.

After losing the first two games of the tournament and the Hawks' new season, we were ready to party and let off some steam. At some point Bev and I found ourselves in a quiet spot among the madness and ended up sitting in the living room and talking through the night. She was an interesting girl and quite smart, but only 19 and fresh out of high school, and unfortunately the vision I had of opening my front door and seeing the house ransacked always loomed close in the back of my mind. So, for the moment at least, I trusted no-one. I was not looking forward to going through another emotional ringer again. That vision stayed with me for a lot of years. But was Fate spinning the dial on me again? Perhaps.

Before ball season had started, the three of us had sat down to come up with a design that would suit the new style of wheeling and take advantage of the new rules that came out of Holland.

While it was Doug's job to build the chair, I was responsible for getting funding to pay for the build. Billy's job was to hound Doug to keep the progress of building the chair going, and to hound me about getting a sponsor. We would all work together to get them assembled.

Once we had the design for the new chair down on paper we decided to make as many of the chair's components out of T6061 aircraft aluminum. Super strong and super light. This choice of material became our first headache because not every welder can work on aluminum. If you heat it up too much it will essentially melt away and it's expensive.

Since we were working on the project with no funding, we had to be careful where we spent our money. We tried a few welding places to inquire about a quote, but they were always out of our price range.

In the meantime, we began to measure out each section of the chair, and since the three of us were different sized athletes, all three chairs would be one-offs. Each piece had to be measured and cut separately.

Instead of two side rails, we decided to build the first ever T-frame racing chair. We wanted it built with one large diameter tube welded underneath a box-like seat, and have the front end welded to the front of the tube. We intended to make custom forks for the new set of 8" front wheels that had just become available on the market and join them together with a custom tie-rod set up.

We had already experienced breaking off a rear axle and realized that with our back wheels cambered out even farther, a lot of stress was going to be put on the inside bearings and the axles. While the wheels on a bicycle are supported by forks on both sides of the hub that help equal out the stress on the axle, the rear axles take a lot of stress on a racing chair. If we could relieve the pressure on the inside bearing, would the chair glide better?

We intended to mill custom hubs out of solid pieces of aluminum, using two different sized bearings; a much larger diameter bearing for the inside of the hub and a smaller bearing on the outside. Tapered axles milled twice the thickness of regular axles would slide into the finished hub. The hub would be extended a couple of inches past the spokes and threaded.

Hand-rims were typically attached to the rear wheels by 4 or 5 metal straps that were welded to the inside of the rim and then attached to the inside of the rear wheel rim. Our idea was to make hand-rims that spun on and off the wheel hub instead, so we could have different sizes to choose from until we found the optimum size for each of our applications.

We wanted the hand-rims built with a threaded centre hub, with 3 aluminum arms welded to the inside. A threaded aluminum cap with a keyway would screw onto the end of the hub to keep everything tight. The hubs would be threaded in opposite directions so that the force of pushing on the hand-rims would keep them tight on the hubs, and the keyway would prevent them coming off in our hands when we attempted to stop by grabbing the rims.

The finished products were a thing of beauty and a testament to Doug's skill on the lathe since he milled 3 sets of rear hubs from solid blocks of aluminum, as well as tapered axles that fit like a glove and threaded caps to finish off the rear wheels.

However, this took months, and we still hadn't found a welding solution. Eventually, Doug decided he would take a course and learn how to MIG and TIG weld and we would fabricate the chairs ourselves. However, he was not into "going to school" so he bought himself a few books on welding instead. He taught himself the skill with some borrowed equipment, but all of this took time, and we were way behind schedule before we were into the new year.

Over the years, as we tried to stabilize our legs and control our balance leaning forward, everyone realized that bracing the knees higher helped prevent you from falling forward past your balance point. You only wanted to lean forward far enough to enable yourself to get a full arm extension, but still give yourself room be able to raise yourself up enough to prepare for the next stroke.

Chapter 10: House of Cards

In the early '80s, this was accomplished by stabilizing one leg on a strap and crossing the other leg over. The bottom foot was then raised inch by inch until the athlete found the sweet spot. High enough that you would not fall forward to the point that you lost your balance, but low enough that you were not prevented from getting full extension on your downward stroke. Eventually we realized that raising both legs was more efficient but for a year at least, many racers crossed their legs.

Since one of the major differences between all the classes was the degree of impairment in the abdominal muscles, this small change in the seating position made the athletes in the lower classes suddenly much faster and more competitive against the higher classes. By decreasing the need for your abdominals to play such a large part in your overall performance, it became a huge step moving forward. Everyone was getting faster, especially the quad racers who had no working abdominal muscles at all.

This seating position also had another added benefit, perhaps equally as important. By lifting the legs higher, the feet were now closer to the body. This took pressure off the short front end of the chair and its glide ability improved greatly. We began to realize that the energy we were generating was being forced downward, instead of out in front, and that's why our chairs were coasting a lot less farther than they should have.

Sometimes you had to change your seating in the chair to ensure your shoulders were in the proper position to push on the rims, but the difference in body stability and the ability to generate power was noticeable. Years later we would come to realize that the longer the front of your chair was, the better its ability to glide and top speed would increase dramatically. But for now, the front wheels stayed where they were.

Chapter 11:
Year of The Disabled

In February of '81 the Variety Village Sports Training and Fitness Centre was officially opened in Scarborough. This was a state-of-the-art facility built for the disabled youth of Ontario and it continues to inspire to this day. Untold hundreds of disabled kids have come to Variety, and not only learned sport skills, but the even harder skill of navigating life as a disabled kid, with its unique challenges and pitfalls.

For myself, and all the other veteran racers in Southern Ontario, it afforded us the opportunity to train all year long and not have to rely on basketball to keep our fitness levels up. Plus, for the kids working out in the facility, we were tangible evidence that if you trained, you could do amazing things with enough hard work.

For years, Variety had indoor track meets in January and March and the facility would eventually host competitions at nearby Birchmount Stadium in conjunction with able-bodied track organizations. While these competitions were usually limited to athletes from Southern Ontario, over the years more and more world-class racers trained at Variety before leaving for an international competition, especially when Graham became Sports Director at the facility. I am so proud, humbled and honored to have a spot on the Variety Village Wall of Fame. Being inducted was the greatest moment in my racing life.

With the arrival of spring, we were not far along in the building process. Money was still hard to come by but eventually we managed to find a place with a lathe and welding equipment that we could afford to rent for a few months.

Chapter 11: Year of The Disabled

Then the build went into overdrive, and when it was all said and done, we had two days to spare before the first ever regionals in Peterborough were upon us.

With not much training under our belts due to long hours in the shop, it showed in our slow times. Nonetheless, the chairs felt comfortable and went around the corners smoothly. Now the hard work would begin. Time to get in shape.

My slalom race produced much better results. Ever since the games in Rio, I had been busy experimenting with different frames and wheel combinations. When I returned from Brazil, the first thing I did was buy a pair of 20" bicycle rims and tires, but when my personal life got complicated, I never did get around to having hand-rims made. Now that I had an apartment and a job, not to mention that Bev and I had been dating for more than a year, I was slowly getting into a better frame of mind and the urge to compete again had risen to the surface.

One day I was catching some sun in the park out front of the Co-op, when I saw a kid go flying by on his mountain bike. And suddenly I had a great idea. I went to a local bike shop to see what they had in stock. They had all the regular stuff, but they also catered to the mountain bike crowd and had a great range of custom wheels. I told them what I had in mind, and I soon left with a pair of 20" gold alloy 2" wide mountain bike rims, and a pair of red, knobby off-road tires.

I intended to push off the tires instead of having hand-rims. The wide bike rims, combined with the fat mountain bike tires were much more stable than the regular 20" rims I bought the year before, and without the hand-rims, they gave me the added benefit of an extra two inches of clearance on both sides of the chair. They were comfortable and with gloves, they gave me a good grip. I felt it would help tremendously going through the many slalom gates.

On the course during the regionals, I was correct on all counts and the near completed chair worked perfectly. It still needed some work on the footplates before the provincials rolled around but getting the newly dubbed 'SBS' racing chairs ready for the Scarborough Nationals took priority.

While the build of the racing chair was still ongoing, I answered the phone at work one day, and the call was from Spar Aerospace. They were a hi-tech

Toronto company that designed, tested and built parts for NASA's space shuttle development program. They had read an article in the newspaper about me trying to get funding for our new chairs and they wondered if I would be interested in having them build me a prototype racing frame. While our build was finally reaching completion, I was not going to turn down the offer, and decided to go to their facility to see what they had in mind.

I was met by Frank Mee, the design laboratory supervisor, and we talked about the chair. He took measurements from my old racer and told me he would get back to me with a prototype.

When Terry Fox arrived in Thunder Bay the previous September, no-one realized that the Marathon of Hope had come to an end. Everyone was stunned to learn that cancer had reappeared, and he was flown back to BC for treatment. On June 28th, just 9 months later, he passed away.

Fast forward to today and the name Terry Fox rings as loudly as before. The Terry Fox Run is still held every September, but not just in Canada anymore. Now the world celebrates his courage and determination as the fight against one of man's worst enemies continues.

The three of us were pumped with excitement when we finally rolled the 'SBS' racers out onto the track for the Ontario Games in Burlington. They were quite the topic and drew a lot of attention throughout the weekend's races. All aluminum, they were the De Lorean's of the racetrack. I couldn't wait to test them out under duress.

For me, the ability to launch the chair off the line quickly turned out to be its best feature, by far. My knee positioning was perfect. With my legs crossed, I could rest my chest on my knee, and get the chair moving effortlessly.

I was still untouchable in the 100, but my lack of fitness still caught up to me as the distances lengthened. I knew from just the little amount of time I had spent in the chair, that I would be rolling a lot faster once my fitness level matched the chairs potential, but at that moment I was not in the best of shape. I still needed to tweak my sitting position in the chair before Scarborough as well, but they worked good enough for the three of us to make the provincial team.

Chapter 11: Year of The Disabled

I wasn't happy with the footplates on my slalom chair during the regionals, and I was not quite finished modifying the platform by the time the provincials arrived. My lack of legal footplates got me disqualified as a result, but boy did I work my way through the course in record time. The extra space the new set-up gave me, provided ample room between the gates. I was looking forward to doing the slalom as well as racing in Scarborough.

The only thing I wasn't prepared for was getting let go from my job a couple of weeks before the nationals. The company was moving the business to another facility and did not require as many employees. Would I ever head to the nationals without something coming up?

In July, Variety Village held its 1st 10K road race. It began in front of Variety and went down Danforth Avenue to the stop lights at Birchmount Rd. The course turned right and right again on Pinegrove Avenue, travelled up the hill through a couple of more side streets, until we found ourselves back on the Danforth. From there we raced down the hill to the finish line in front of the Village. I was fortunate enough to hold off the field to win in 31:17.

The new 'SBS' chairs again received a ton of attention when we first rolled onto the Birchmount track for the '81 Canadian Games for the Physically Disabled in Scarborough. The cameras came out and people began taking pictures while we warmed up. As Billy leisurely wheeled along the front straight, an ever-present rules committee member followed him, taking notes. No worries, it was legal. We made sure of that.

I got a great jump at the gun in the 100 and though the field was closing in on me, I held them off for the gold. I managed a bronze in the 400, but it wasn't hard to see that my fitness level was not yet up to par with the competition unfortunately.

The combined 1500 was a super fast race. Quebec's Andre Viger had warmed up by winning the 800 in record time and at the gun for the 1500, he went out fast. Ontario's Ron Robillard attempted to stay with him, but by the time the third lap had begun, he began falling behind. Andre continued to pull away and finished in 4:24.3 well under the existing world record.

As Ron's pace slowed due to his overly fast first laps, I began to close the gap. While he ultimately held me off by 1/10th to claim the silver, in my attempt to reel him in, I finished in 4:54.9 and made good on my personal goal of wheeling under the 5-minute mark. The 'SBS' chair was a success.

As dominant as Andre was, Ontario's Paul Clark was equally unstoppable in the Class 2 events, winning gold in the 100 (20.3), the 200 (39 flat) for a Canadian record, the 400 (1:17.2) under the world record, and two more Canadian records in the 800 and 1500 metres (2:41.0 / 5:13.4). It was no wonder that our combination of Paul, Ron, me and anchor Tim Haslam smashed the old 4 x 400 Canadian relay record, stopping the clock at 4:45.7.

Over on the slalom course, it was good news. With my new footplates attached, the slalom chair was now legal, and the new chair worked perfectly. I wheeled a no-fault run and took back my national slalom crown.

The Pan Am Games were scheduled for next summer in Halifax, and I was hoping to make the team so I could have another head-to-head competition with American Dave Williamson if he was still on the team.

On Sept 9th, Montreal hosted the first sanctioned international wheelchair marathon in Canada. This was an invitation-only field of some of the best wheelers in Canada and the US, assembled to showcase the advancements of wheelchair road racing, and to lobby for more wheelchair divisions to be included in marathons held around the world. Racers also wanted to get the wheelchair marathon included as a medal event at Stoke as well. I was pleasantly surprised when my invitation arrived in the mail. Me doing a marathon. Wow.

Graham figured I was mad to even think of doing such a thing, but since I had every intention of going to Montreal, he made sure I understood that I had to go out slow and build my speed over time. Under no circumstance should I take off and try to stay with anyone in the first few miles, regardless of my fitness level. I needed to get in a nice rhythm and work with anyone who was on the same pace as me. If I went out too fast, I'd burn out before the race was over and he didn't want that to happen.

The race began at the Jacques Cartier Bridge and worked its way through old Montreal, eventually arriving at the Island and onto the Jacques Villeneuve track and the finish line. Rain had made the downhill sections slippery, especially rounding corners in Old Montreal, and so there were a

Chapter 11: Year of The Disabled

couple of racers who crashed but were able to eventually carry on. Those few sections of cobblestone roadway challenged our stability, but mostly it was a good course.

The field was impressive, to say the least. The American team consisted of Paralympians Junior Rice, Marty Ball, and Bob Hall, all experienced wheelchair marathoners. The Canadian contingent was led by Andre Viger, Mel Fitzgerald, Dan Westley and about a dozen more racers from across Canada. The three of us from Ontario that were included in the field had never done a marathon and between Richmond Hill's Tim Haslam, Kitchener's Ron van Elswyk and I, we each wanted to be considered the fastest from Ontario. When the main group surged out at the gun as expected, I tried to pace myself in another group that included Lenny Marriott and Peter Brooks, two marathoners from BC.

In the end, to the surprise of more than a few I expect, John Lundie of Manitoba held off Mel Fitzgerald and won the first Montreal Marathon, finishing in 2:07:20. Mel crossed the line in 2:09:37. Andre was third in 2:13:19. I ended up in 13th place, in 2:38:32 and finished strong.

I realized that I could have pushed myself harder sooner and gotten a faster time once I saw that there was only a couple of miles to go, but it really was better than struggling to finish. I realized, regardless of my time compared to the serious marathoners, I was able to wheel the twenty-six plus miles it took to complete the race. While there was obviously room for improvement, I was pleased with the outcome. I was now a marathoner. Both Ron and Tim finished in just under 3 hours.

Having done the Montreal Marathon less than a month before, I decided that I wanted to do my hometown marathon and so I signed up for the 4th Annual Labatt's Toronto Marathon, set to run early that October. My basketball teammate, Brien Foran had just begun racing and only had 10K runs under his belt, but he decided to race the marathon as well.

There was no wheelchair division of course, since I didn't think to contact Paul Poce, the race co-ordinator to give him a heads-up that we planned to enter. I hoped if we showed well, he would explore the possibility of including a wheelchair division the following year.

The course had us heading out from Queens's Park, where we raced south on University Ave to Queen St. We turned right and headed west to

Kipling Avenue, eventually making our way north to Bloor St, where we headed east and into Varsity Stadium with a crowd of 3,000 to cheer us on to the finish line.

The racecourse itself did pose a few problems that we encountered along the way, however. We had to navigate a foot path for one stretch of the race and had to jump up and down a couple of curbs in other places. The worst section proved to be the streetcar tracks on Queen St. I thought I might ditch a couple of times but slowing down got me through those rough spots.

I finished in 2:47:01, good for 96th overall, in a race won by New Zealand runner Kevin Ryan. As the first wheelchair winner, I got a lot of good coverage, before during and after the race. While the course kept me from setting a faster time than Montreal, my hope was that we made a good enough impression to warrant our own wheelchair division the following year.

We were well received by our fellow competitors and got lots of encouragement from both the runners, officials and spectators that we met during the event. Going downhill runners would ask for a ride, and I'd say, "No problem, just as long as I can hang onto your shorts on the way back up".

After the marathon was over, I was contacted a few days later, by Jerry Mandel, President of Speedy Muffler King, and Bob McTavish VP of Corp. Development. They were interested in sponsoring me to compete in next year's Boston Marathon and help fund our racing chairs. It was the break we needed.

"Although disabled, Toronto marathoner Chris Stoddart will be able to compete in the 1982 Boston Marathon. Capping its 25th Anniversary celebrations, Speedy Muffler King has announced it will underwrite a racing chair, designed and built by Chris, and his two partners, and his travelling expenses to the premier event.

"Our 25 years of growth and success have been a result of our meeting and beating many challenges," he said, when making the announcement. "We felt that Stoddart's remarkable will to succeed, was in keeping with ours. Speedy's support of Stoddart is a tribute to his competitive spirit".

I had my first big sponsor, and I was determined to make them proud.

By now, I was not the only wheelchair athlete living in the David B. Archer Co-op. Along with future Paralympian teammate Bob Ellery, both

Chapter 11: Year of The Disabled

long-time friends Marv and Brien had found apartments in the building as well. Doug and Hawk teammates Dennis Kloppenburg and John Klis lived nearby as well, and those of us who raced got in the habit of meeting at the Co-op and wheeling out to Cherry Beach for our road workouts and then cruising the Boardwalk before racing back to the Esplanade.

I did most of my formal training on the track at Central Tech High School, and by now we had lots of company since it was where the Spitfires trained as well. The club had grown into a big organization, and its members were not limited to just playing basketball anymore. A great number of their players competed in other sports, especially wheelchair racing. Many of the guys I trained with, lined up beside me at provincial and national competitions. Daryl Taylor, Mike Blackned, Angela Ieriti, and Spitfire's Dave Lash and Mike O'Brien were only a few that trained on this downtown track. Almost everyone trained here until the snow began and then we headed indoors to Variety.

Before the new ball season began, Spitfire's Mike Bryce offered me the opportunity to play on one of their SOWBL teams, so I joined the Spitfires organization and played on the Shooting Stars with Jerry Tonello as my coach. I met all the players and hit it off right away with a guy named Gino Vendetti. This was to be my first experience with the concept of "six degrees of separation".

Gino explained that he was born with cerebral palsy and was given up at birth. He was raised by a couple named Johnson, that took in many disabled children, and they had a place on Cook's Bay, the southernmost bay on Lake Simcoe. He went through a lot of operations, many more than I had to endure, and he got picked on a lot by the surrounding kids that came up on weekends to the cottages that were spread around the bay. The only person that was always nice to him was a girl around the same age named Bev Waddell. Are you kidding me?

The first time Bev came over to my apartment, I started up a conversation about her grandmother's cottage on Cook's Bay. Didn't you say there was a disabled kid named Gino Johnson that you knew? I kept my new teammate's story out of the conversation, but I invited her to go with me to see Mike again and to meet some of my new teammates on the Spitfires. The following week she came with me to practise.

I worked my way through the team introducing Bev until I came to Gino. What a laugh. Both their eyes got the same look at the same time. Gino…? Bev…? What were the odds? We all had a great laugh, and they had a great conversation catching up after a decade of not seeing each other. I had a big smile on my face, and was kidding when I said, "Just remember, you had your chance. She's mine now."

Another coincidence to the story is that Gino got involved in wheelchair sports after seeing me on television with Mr. Spock and listening to me talk about wheelchair basketball and all the other sports that were available. It really is a small world.

Unfortunately, joining the Spitfire organization to play in the SOWBL did not go over well with some of my teammates on the Hawks. Some of the guys still felt slighted when they were not asked to join the Spitfires when they were first formed and didn't like the idea of my playing with them in the NWBA, and then playing on the Shooting Stars against them in the SOWBL. So, despite making the Conference All-Star team at the end of the season, I was informed that I was not welcome on the Hawks anymore, and only played with them for a couple of seasons.

Just after the Scarborough Games finished in August, Spar Aerospace had dropped off the prototype frame for me to check out. Unlike the 'SBS' chair, this frame was the bare minimum. Unfortunately, certain dimensions used to manufacture the prototype had been incorrect and the back wheels didn't fit, so with the 'SBS' chair up and running, the frame sat idle.

But the Scarborough Games had opened my eyes to new ideas. I really liked the chair that BC's Dan Westley had been racing in. Being a double amputee and not having to worry about the placement of his legs, it allowed him the opportunity to have the least amount of metal in which to build his frame from. And while I was not an amputee, I did have short legs that were light and flexible enough so that I could situate them where I wanted.

I decided to try the minimalistic route and fished out the Spar frame. It looked much like Dan's chair, and a lot more simplistic than the 'SBS' chair that we had just built. It would still require some fabrication before I could

Chapter 11: Year of The Disabled

use it to race in, and even though it would cost me more money, I decided that two chairs were better than one.

I took it to a new wheelchair company in Toronto, Canadian Wheelchair Manufacturing, where I explained what I needed done. I wanted to keep the same rear wheels with the custom 'SBS' hubs and spin-on hand-rims, but I wanted the front wheels closer together and without a tie-rod system.

While the 'SBS' racer turned out to be a one-year wonder, even after everything we put into its manufacture, this new chair I dubbed the 'Rail', worked well for years until I was forced into the next step.

Now that disabled competitions in Canada had been recognized as true sporting events, and we were being tested for banned substances, like the able-bodied athletes were, we were happy when it was announced that we would be eligible for financial assistance under the new Disabled Sports Athlete Assistance Program. This carding criteria would remain in effect until the 1984 Paralympics and had the following qualifications that had to be met.

The event you were competing in must have a minimum of 15 entries from 10 different countries. An A-card was issued to athletes who had placed 1st, 2nd or 3rd in recent international competition and a B-card for athletes who had placed 4th, 5th or 6th.

My B-card enabled me to receive $250.00 in the spring and another $250 in the fall towards equipment or travel expenses. Not a lot of money, but it was a start. If nothing else, I hoped the money would keep me in high-pressure tires for the year.

Chapter 12: Penalty Free

Ontario wheelchair racing history was made in April '82 when the Hamilton International Marathon was designated as Ontario's Wheelchair Marathon Championships. Since there were not a lot of athletes that first year, it was an Open Class race. Wheeling in the 'Rail', I rolled in second behind new kid on the block, Class 4 Chris Daw. My time of 2:39:39 was faster than I wheeled Toronto last year, but Montreal remained my fastest time for now.

I had hoped to wheel in the Boston Marathon that year, but I failed to realize that there were qualifying standards, and I didn't have a fast enough marathon time to qualify for the race. I was hoping to rectify that situation in the future.

At the regionals, the 'Rail' proved I made the right choice. It was very quick off the line, resulting in a personal best in the 100 metres of 17.5 seconds. The rest of my races were close to personal bests as well. This was a good sign since the next step would be the Training Camp in Halifax on the track where the Pan American Wheelchair Games scheduled for August at St. Mary's University, would be held.

And as it turned out, the June training camp in Halifax was a good week with lots of quality workouts and a chance to do any fine tuning to our chairs. I felt a lot stronger and faster than I had been in years and I was looking forward both to the track races as well as unveiling my new slalom chair.

Back home in Ontario, I ran the table at the 8th Ontario Games in Sarnia. I was as ready as I was going to be.

Chapter 12: Penalty Free

Before the Pan Am Games began, Variety Village and Birchmount Stadium hosted the 1st Integrated Track and Field Classic in Canada on August 8th, featuring an international field of world class runners and wheelchair racers that would try to break the 4-minute Metric Mile.

These were not Class by Class races, that were the norm in our sport. With the advancement of technology that was narrowing the gap among the disability classes, Open Class races were becoming more and more prevalent.

I was second in the 100-metre showdown, getting nipped at the line by Alberta's Ron Minor, who set a new Class 4 record by winning in 17.2. to my 17.5.

Ron's teammate from Edmonton, Ron Payette won both the open 400 and 800 races. A cancer research specialist, he went under the Class 3 record in both races, winning the 400 in 1:10.4 and the 800 in 2:24.10. He was ready for Halifax as well.

Both had come to Variety to train under Graham, leading up to Halifax in August and Ron Minor was quoted as saying: "Most important and best decision I ever made concerning sports. There is no coach in Canada to match Graham Ward."

It was an epic battle of Class 5 racers in the featured race, as BC's Dan Westley won the Metric Mile over NFLD's Mel Fitzgerald in a thrilling race that came down to less than an inch and produced the first sub-4-minute mile in our sports history. Dan stopped the clock at 3:58.05 with Mel 2/100th of a second behind. I clocked in at 4:51.4, a personal best and good for 5th.

In the featured able-bodied Metric Mile, Kenyan Sosphenes Bitok finished in 3:52.5. Paul Steed of Toronto was second in 3:59.6. This was the fastest mile in years on Canadian soil.

As well, Toronto's Dave Reid ran a 4:03 mile and broke Bruce Kidd's long-standing Canadian junior record.

The last two weeks before Halifax were spent fine tuning things and making sure everything was ready for the Pan Am's. I was getting more comfortable wheeling in the 'Rail', and I was itching to see how my new slalom chair would match up against Mr. Williamson if he was part of the US team.

After the less-than-ideal conditions we were forced to adapt to in Rio at the '78 Pan Am Games, we knew going into Halifax that this competition would be well organized, with great accommodations and devoid of the security issues that we faced in Brazil. Having already been housed at St. Mary's University for our training camp a month earlier, we were confident that we would be comfortable, well fed, and as a bonus, us track guys were literally able to roll out the front door of the residence and onto the Huskies track.

The Games ran from Aug 21-29 and had been well publicized in the months leading up to the opening ceremonies and so it was no surprise to find the stands full every day, regardless of the weather conditions. The opening ceremonies were excellent, and Team Hostess Colleen Craig carried the big Maple Leaf flag, while Dan Westley and I led the Canadian contingent around the Huskies Stadium track. Let the Games begin.

As is usually the case at the Pan Am Games, the American track team would be our biggest challenge. Even though a few of the South American countries featured world class wheelers, only the US team had more depth and a much higher level of chair technology.

Going into the competition, the focus, in Canada at least, had centred on Rick Hansen and his recent success on the wheelchair marathon circuit, having won the famed Miami Marathon in April in 2:05:54 and winning the Canadian Wheelchair Marathon Championship in May.

Coverage was also centred on Class 5 racers Mel Fitzgerald of St. John's Newfoundland and Surrey BC's Dan Westley.

While all the various events drew crowds to watch us compete, none were larger than when we were racing on the track. Wheelchair racing was then, as is now, one of the premiere events for spectators, from my point of view, of course. This competition could be looked upon as our team's coming out party.

Unfortunately, the weather proved to be a factor throughout the week as rain and high winds were the norm for the competition. Its effects did not seem to bother the power pushers as track records began to fall on the first day, but it was proving to be a problem for myself.

The 'Rail' was the lightest racer I had ever wheeled in and being a good twenty or so pounds lighter than my competitors, the wind was playing havoc

Chapter 12: Penalty Free

with my ability to stay in my lane as I went around the first corner, and it was acting like an invisible roadblock as I headed into it down the backstretch. I needed the wind to die down once the races started or I would be in trouble.

Racing began with the 100 and the team got off to a good start. Andre Viger won the Class 3 gold in Pan Am record time while I lost the bronze by a foot. An uncharacteristically slow reaction time in the final cost me a chance at a medal.

Rick won the Class 4 gold in the world record time of 17.5, over American veteran Jim Knaub, with Ron Minor wheeling in for bronze

Dan Westley held off Dean Barrett of the US in winning the Class 5 event in the world record time of 16.10.

First thing on the agenda Tuesday was the 400 heats and finals. Heats took up most of the morning since there was usually a good number of athletes competing in the shorter races.

It was soon apparent during my 400 heat that going against the wind was going to be a major concern for me if the conditions did not change. The wind was gusting to the point that when I went around the corner, it threatened to tip me over. I struggled mightily on the backstretch until I turned the corner for home. With the wind behind me I did pick up speed, but ultimately, I found myself just making the Class 3 final

It was the same conditions when we lined up for all the marbles. I was in Lane 2 with everyone out in front of me except for the one athlete to the left. The gun sounded and I got a good jump and was picking up speed when the wind pushed the front of my chair towards the centre of the track. Luckily, I stayed in my lane but by the time I had corrected myself and went around the corner and straight into the wind I was in last. All I could do was put my head down and push for all I was worth.

Andre and George Murray of the US battled out in front until the end when Andre finished ahead in 1:09.5. American John Rodolph won the bronze. I was 7th at the head of the stretch but with the wind behind me, I got close to a medal but still had to settle for 4th.

Rick edged Jim Knaub of the US in the world record time of 1:05.4 in winning the Class 4 final. Ron Minor won the bronze.

In a thrilling Class 5 final, Dan nipped Mel (1:04.6/1:05.3). Dean Barrett of the US was third. All three were under the existing world record.

Later in the day I was hoping to get on the podium when I wheeled the slalom, but by late afternoon, it was so windy and with the rain coming down, it made it unsafe to climb the ramp that was part of the course. It was postponed until the Wednesday, but when Wednesday arrived, it was cancelled again. The 10 Premiers were scheduled to make an appearance on the Thursday, so it was put off once again. But I was ready when they were.

With an off day on Wednesday, the weather had eased off a bit on the Thursday for the early 800 metre races. The rain stopped and the wind died down. Unfortunately, I was not able to take advantage of the better weather, since I did not enter the event, having chosen the slalom instead. But the team added 3 more gold and a couple of silvers once all the races were completed.

Andre continued to roll, winning Class 3 gold in 2:19.5. Rick's 2:12.6 was under the existing world record, and good for another gold in Class 4.

Mel, Dan and Kris Lenzo of the US put on their own show in the Class 5 final. It was Fitzgerald's turn to win gold (2:12.9) over Westley (2:13.4). Lenzo garnered the bronze.

Thursday also featured the 200 finals, and I was feeling a lot better since I knew the wind would be at my back for a change and that would help more than hamper. The 200 turned out to be my best race of the competition and the most aggravating, all at the same time.

I timed my start perfectly and I was rolling and out with the lead as the wind began to push me around the corner and onto the top of the stretch. I still had the lead about ¾ of the way down the stretch when Andre and the athlete from Mexico began to close the gap. They both came close, but they didn't catch me. I won by less than an inch. I was super happy since this was the first time, I had beaten Andre on the track.

But wait, somehow bib numbers got switched after the race, and when the dust had settled, I had been bumped to bronze. I told Graham for certain that neither one of them beat me to the finish line, and the protest and re-evaluation of the pictures changed my result from bronze to silver, but I was still ticked off. To this day, this race still aggravates me.

Meanwhile, Class 4 gold went to Rick in the world record time of 32.4 and Ron Minor pocketed the silver, clocking in at 33.5.

Chapter 12: Penalty Free

Both Mel and Dan were not entered in the Class 5 200, but Toronto's Dave Lash won a bronze to add to Canada's total.

Randy Dueck of Winnipeg won his second silver in the 1B 200 final.

Rick's gold in the 200 was the team's 46th medal and broke the record for the most medals won by a Canadian team in international competition. The record of 45 medals was formerly held by the '78 Canadian Commonwealth Games team competing in Edmonton.

Finally, it was time for the slalom, something that I had been eagerly anticipating. I had a completely different chair than the one I used for the slalom in Rio, and I was hoping I had found the best combination.

When we built the 'SBS' chair in 1981, I used the racing chair frame that E & J had built for me in '75 for the slalom. It was the same chair I used in Rio. The Spitfires found me another basketball chair frame when I joined the team, and the first time I tried it with the 20" rear wheels, I knew the solid frame was an improvement over my old folding version.

Set up along the 100-metre straightaway in front of the packed grandstand, it was going to be fun. As usual the race consisted of a series of obstacles that each athlete had to manoeuvre through. Over time the slalom course was standardized to prevent surprises by overly enthusiastic slalom designers and to allow for a record time to be established.

As I had hoped, veteran US athlete Dave Williamson was on the American team. He had won the gold back in '78 and I remember him smiling at me and venturing that I might have given him a run for the gold if I hadn't gone the wrong way! It was all in fun, since Dave was one of the classiest athletes I ever competed against, but I still wanted to return the favour.

When I saw him during the opening ceremonies, I was riding in my new slalom chair. A sneak peek to show him I hadn't been idle since Rio, and I was ready for a rematch.

The media was all set up as we visually went through the course in preparation. Again, you could look the course over, but you still could not execute any of the manoeuvres in front of you. This was a good set-up. No surprises like you find sometimes. Just normal obstacles in whatever order the organizers had felt like putting together that would showcase our speed and dexterity.

As luck would have it, I drew an early number. I like being one of the first to go. Done well, it gives the rest of the field something to think about. Touching a pylon in your haste to beat my time could be your downfall.

I wheeled a smooth-as-silk race. No missed gates and I touched nothing. Up and down the ramp with a 360 degree turn on top, through the gates, under the bar and a quick dash to the finish line. He still won the silver though, with Juan Silva of Brazil taking home the bronze. My 59 second elapsed time was the quickest of all the classes.

Dave was gracious in defeat, as I knew he would be, and he hoped that we could have the rubber match in Illinois, the site of the '84 Paralympics.

I was not the only Canadian that competed in the slalom though. Teammates Julien Wedge won the Class 1B race and Ed Batt did the same in the 1C final.

Saturday was the 5,000, the longest of all the races offered and this was another distance where the Canadian team dominated. Andre won the Class 3 race (15:14.8), Rick captured the Class 4 event (14:26.9) for a world record and Mel capped in off with a gold in Class 5 (14:32.8) for a world record of his own. Lennie Mariotte of BC captured the Class 5 silver in 15:20.6.

The 1500 is always an exciting race, and the Sunday finals were no exception. Based on how my chair was reacting in the heavy wind, Graham thought I should tuck behind someone going against the wind and make any moves when the wind was behind me.

At the gun, the field began to spread out and headed down the back stretch in single file, with me near the end of the line. It stayed that way until the next lap. I don't know who initiated contact, but suddenly the athlete in front of me veered to the outside. Luckily, I did the same, and went around the wreck, which, unfortunately included Andre.

On the last lap, with the wind behind me, I overtook a couple of racers and came away with the bronze. Good strategy paid off.

In the Class 4 final, Rick continued to be unbeatable, winning the 1500 in world record time (4:13.3) and Dan won gold over Mel in world record time (4:08.80 / 4:08.81) to claim the Class 5 crown.

The only thing left to decide was who would win the relays, and as it is with the regular Olympics, the relays are the cherries on top of the cake.

Chapter 12: Penalty Free

With all the medals that the team had accumulated throughout the week, we felt we were the team to beat.

However, it wasn't hard to see that I was easily the weakest link in the chain as we got ready for the 4 x 100 metre relay. Since Andre did more distance racing, and even though he won the 100 earlier, he was entered in the 4 x 200 and 4 x 400 metre relays. As a sprinter, the 4 x 100 was mine this time around.

My strength was always my start off the line, so I figured all I had to do was get a good start, go around the corner, tag Rick and the guys would take care of the rest. My only concern was still the wind. A 30-knot headwind up the backstretch was not going to help me get around the corner but there was no way to prevent it, so I hoped it wouldn't affect me too much going forward.

I got my usual good start but as I picked up speed going around the corner, the wind threatened to push me straight, and that effectively killed my momentum. I struggled mightily to touch Rick. By the time I had tagged him, we were behind, by a lot.

Rick and then Ron Minor powered their way up the backstretch into the headwind and around the bend. Dan flew down the straight to the finish line. But even his blinding speed was not enough to make up for my deficiency. Four teams made the final and we were in fourth.

There was no question where the problem lay, and as the wind just continued to blow, an attempt was made to make a substitution. As I said, even though Andre rarely wheeled the 100, he was strong enough to overcome the wind and give the team a much better chance.

Graham took me aside to explain the situation. This is the final track day and there are dignitaries, and a full crowd here to watch Rick win more gold medals...etc. Didn't have to tell me, I knew as much. There was no way I could overcome that wind, and unless it died down before the afternoon's finals, I'd be the guy that cost us a medal, never mind not winning the gold. Word came down substitutions were only allowed in case of injury, and since I was fine, the request was denied. So, there it was, me or nothing.

Never in all my years of racing, have I agonized about a race so much beforehand. I looked for some magic elixir that would somehow get me through the wind. Too bad for me if I didn't win a medal but losing one that 3 teammates were counting on your contribution to make happen, weighed heavy on my mind.

And then the answer came to me! I had an idea and I rushed to find Graham. After I told him my plan, he said to gather the guys together and make my pitch. So, I rounded the guys up and I said, "listen, I know I'm the weak link here and I know it goes against what is normally done, but I think I need to wheel the anchor. I am just not strong enough to overcome this wind and my chair is being moved about as I wheel. Dan is strong enough to cut through the wind and if we have a lead right away, I don't see us being overtaken. Once I get rolling, the wind is going to help blow me down the straight like a leaf across a parking lot."

Rick thought about it for a few moments and then said, "Well we're not going to win the way it is, so if Dan is willing to switch places, It's fine by me." I knew Dan would agree. His team first attitude would have him gladly switch places if it meant we had a better chance of winning. With his blessing we lined up for the final.

As expected, at the gun, Dan bolted us into a first-quarter lead, slicing through the wind like a knife through butter and rounding the corner to tag Rick with no problem. Trouble flared at the next exchange when Ron miss-judged how fast Rick was coming towards him and left too soon. He had to slow his momentum down to ensure he did not go past the takeover zone before being tagged. We lost ground.

Of course, this just amped Ron up even more and he muscled his way around the corner to make up for lost time. Our team was wheeling in lanes 3 and 4 and with the Americans in lanes 1 and 2, I could see both Ron and the US racer, coming around the corner towards me. The American anchor, Dean Barrett, had already been tagged and was picking up speed as he raced towards me, when Ron reached out and touched my shoulder. This is one of just a few races that I can close my eyes and see it unfold in slow-motion.

As soon as Ron touched me, I let 'er fly. Technique went out the window. I sat upright, out of my usual tuck and began to fan my wheels as fast as I could. The wind caught me, and I was gone.

With the Canadian team stationed just past the finish line to the right, I could see them cheering me on, and when I crossed the line, I held up

Chapter 12: Penalty Free

my index finger as I coasted around the bend and into the wind. We had pulled it off.

What a great victory lap that was. I was so happy it turned out the way it did. After that heavy headwind had prevented me from getting better results all week, that day the wind became my friend, for one event at least. Later in the afternoon, with Andre on board, the guys won both the 4 x 200 and 4 x 400 metre relays to cap off a tremendous week of racing.

With these Games complete, everyone's sight was set on the '84 Paralympics, slated for the University of Illinois.

Back home, with track done for the season, we took to the roads once more. Most of our big-name racers were beginning to spend more time competing in marathons and road races down in the United States. With sponsorships, they were able to train and race down south and in Europe during the winter months. The rest of us had to be content with entering any races that we could find to compete in until the snow fell, and then we were back on the hardcourt or on the track at Variety Village.

I wanted to do a marathon prior to the Toronto race, and I finally settled on the Skylon International Marathon in Niagara Falls, scheduled for the end of September. This marathon turned out to be one of the hardest and demanding marathons I ever competed in.

The race ran along the Niagara River starting from the Skylon Observation tower and headed east toward Toronto. It was already quite cold to begin with, but right before the gun sounded to start the race, the wind began to pick up considerably

Soon after, it began to sleet, and the pack was forced to head straight into the wind, and the driving rain. There were few turns or hills in this race, but it was a monumental struggle to continue battling the wind as we inched toward the finish line.

It took me over 3 hours to finally reach the tape, stopping the clock at 3:06:0. It was the slowest marathon time I ever recorded.

Everyone's chair was coated in ice and adding to the ordeal was the fact that the changing area was a wide-open tent that everyone crammed into. Sitting on the cold wet grass while we attempted to change out of our soaking wet clothes for warm ones was not fun.

Ultimately, we waited another hour or so before the awards ceremony started, only to receive this tiny plaque for our efforts, after everything was said and done. Driving home to Toronto through the continuing snowfall was the icing on the cake. I had a week to recover before the Toronto Marathon.

The 5th Labatt's Toronto Marathon was scheduled for early October, and when we still did not have our own division, I voiced my displeasure at the oversight and because of this I was invited to write my views about the marathon and what part the wheelchair athlete should play in the event.

I talked Brien and Marv into entering the race as well, hoping more numbers in the field would help organizers decide that a wheelchair division would be worth the effort. The first leg saw the field heading down University Avenue again.

Positioned in the front row with hundreds of runners all around you, was not for the faint of heart though. If we wanted a wheelchair division in the future, we had to make sure there were no mishaps, and it would not be easy with this setup.

The surge of runners at the gun had them running around us and heading down the street, but once we picked up speed and began to overtake them, we had to be extra careful to go wide and let them know we were passing. Once everyone spread out, we had room to manoeuvre, and we could relax. An incident-free start was extremely important.

We still had to contend with more of those pesky streetcar tracks as we crossed Queen St, and that required us to slow down and cross carefully before picking up the pace once more. Unfortunately, the Toronto Marathon was hardly ever planned out with concerns for the wheelchair division in mind. However, I had a good race and set a personal best in 2:28:33. and good for 12th place overall.

Once October arrived, basketball was in full swing, and one weekend the Spitfire team flew out to Saskatchewan for a weekend tournament featuring the Saskatchewan Cyclones, the Edmonton Northern Lights, Manitoba Golden Ramblers, and the Calgary Grizzlies. Mike sent a small team for the tournament, consisting of Flo Aukema, Bob Bryce, Jerry Tonello, Dave Lash, Les Lam, Mike Holt, Randy Critch and me.

Chapter 12: Penalty Free

We played the Cyclones first and won 60-24. Blowout wins over the Northern Lights (71-36), the Golden Ramblers (58-37) and the Grizzlies (74-19) proved we were unbeatable. The teams had no match for our trio of big guys. Stopping Flo, Jerry or Bob was a tall task, even in a one-on-one situation. Any combination of Flo and Jerry, or Flo and Bob proved unstoppable.

However, during the weekend, I took a lot of flak from the guys I knew on the other teams for playing on a team that relied on their able-bodied players to the extent that we did. Saying that playing with the Spitfires afforded me more opportunities to play more tournaments, instead of just regular season games did nothing to turn down the heat. I had to admit that sitting on the bench for virtually the whole tournament, except for "garbage time" was a little embarrassing considering I was a member of the provincial team.

It wasn't that I disliked the able-bodied playing wheelchair basketball, I just wished as a team we could have seen past our enthusiasm in attempting to promote the able-bodied playing ball, by not having them take such a dominant role. We were not short on players, but it seemed like we got drunk on success and perhaps lost a little perspective.

However, with Jerry as my playing-coach for the time I was a Shooting Star, I certainly learned a lot, as did my teammates. I loved playing basketball for the pure pleasure of playing but Jerry made me focus more and enjoy the experience after the game was over. But I came back home from out West wondering what direction my basketball future would take.

Chapter 13:
A Job for Life

Despite the way the chair reacted in the wind in Halifax, it was light and comfortable, but I was still trying to decide on the best seating position.

By now, everyone sat in their racing chairs in a tucked position, knees elevated with the weight of their legs usually supported by a padded bar under the knees or a strap that your feet rested on. Sometimes a racer would tuck their legs under the seat or position them out in front. It really depended upon your ability to be flexible and the design of your frame.

In Halifax, my legs were anchored out front but nearly all the other racers had their feet resting on a strap below the seat or tucked up underneath. I had experimented with leg placement for years and I felt like as long as my knees were supported, it didn't really matter where my legs were placed. I knew from an aerodynamic point of view that having them out front was the worst set-up of the three choices, but the 'Rail' had no sides and therefore nowhere to place a bar under my knees. To tuck them under me would require welding a bar and two support arms to fit under my knees at the correct height, and I wasn't ready to go that route just yet.

I had ample opportunity to try both set-ups during the winter months while I trained at Variety, and in March I got the opportunity to test both against competition when the facility hosted their 1st Variety Village Indoor track meet.

The event was a great idea and allowed all the kids that trained there, to compete and gain experience racing among themselves. It also afforded them the opportunity to watch the veterans' race and realize that they could be doing the same thing with hard work.

Chapter 13: A Job for Life

Indoors, the 'Rail' worked excellent. Variety's 200-metre track has tight corners and short straights, which meant racing indoors was significantly different that wheeling outside on a regular track. My light front end made it easy to corner with just a twist of my waist and I used that to my advantage. Though competition was usually limited to the wheelies in Southern Ontario, by now we had a good pool of racers in most Classes that competed in the province, so we had some good competitions among ourselves.

I knew my fitness level was high during the 1500 when I wheeled under 5 minutes on the indoor track. It was a first for me and it showed me that I was having no trouble getting around the corners while keeping my speed consistent. For the moment at least, the time was a provincial indoor record.

While Stoke Mandeville still insisted on four wheels, some athletes were bending the rules and beginning to experiment with just one wheel out front. The original idea of the three-wheel racer was the brainchild of Canada's Paul Clark, who began experimenting as far back as 1979.

But by now, he was constructing his own racing chairs from angled aluminum, held together with nuts and bolts. The first time I saw it, it automatically reminded me of the Meccano sets that I used to play with as a kid!

While it wasn't much to look at, it did the job remarkably well. Since it wasn't welded together, parts were interchangeable, and it was perfect for young racers who would soon outgrow a welded frame version. Paul began to sell them as an alternative to the solid frame chair.

Soon he converted his own frame to run a single wheel and raced it in local events. In time, he proved that it was a well made and versatile chair, since it carried him to multiple gold medals before it became obsolete.

Many individuals believed all 3-wheeled racing chairs were prone to crashing during a race, but it was soon disproved, and it wasn't long before many more athletes began experimenting with the 3-wheel concept.

And, while the rule stated that the chair had to have four wheels, there was no mention of size or placement. Sometimes racers would off-set one wheel and mount it so that the wheel just barely touched the surface.

Then athletes began to add the fourth wheel for show. Some went so far as to stick a tiny wheel on the front of their chair like a bobble-head doll sitting on the dashboard of your car! Whatever passed inspection.

But, in the beginning it was a hit and miss proposition. While your chair might be deemed legal at one event, there was no guarantee that it would pass inspection somewhere else.

The Brampton Ontario Games in June was the first step towards my goal of making the '84 Paralympic team. Winning my races and keeping my slalom title, meant I had until August to build on my fitness level and finally decide what my seating position would be. And before I lined up in Sudbury, I had the opportunity to compete in an event close to home.

A week later, still pumped from my race in Toronto, I entered a road race called the Wheels n Heels 15K near Owen Sound. It featured both able-bodied runners and wheelers in a race along Highway 10 from Markdale to Holland Landing. The race was organized to help raise funds for Participation House in Owen Sound.

From Markdale, the field of runners and a half dozen or so of us wheelers headed north toward the finish line in Holland Centre. The course was basically a straight run up and down a series of small hills.

Had a great race with the top runner who paced at about the same speed I did. While he got a lead as we went up the hills, I caught him by the time we got down the other side. This went on for the three of four hills that were on the route. He sprinted up the last hill with about a mile to go and built a good lead.

In the end, he was able to outsprint me to victory, but I had a great time wheeling the race and rolled across in at 40:05. This was a fun race for a good cause.

Our cottage in Buckhorn was not far from the small town of Lindsay, and after reading about the Lindsay 10K Milk Run, I filled out the form on a whim. A good 10k was something I could use to build up my stamina and the chance to wheel with runners was still a new concept for me, so I was looking forward to it. I needed more time in the new chair and I thought this race would be more fun than just wheeling on a track.

The race was in mid-July and naturally, I was the only wheeler, but Bev and I were well received, nonetheless. I liked it so much that I ended up wheeling this race a half dozen years in a row. A couple of times by myself but usually there was at least one or two other wheelers who would race with me.

That first year, the race began with one lap of the town's old dirt horse track, which was a bit difficult to wheel on, as you can imagine. The runners disappeared one by one until I made it onto smooth pavement and began to pick up speed. Once on the road though, it was smooth sailing until we reached the top of Main Street.

From there it was a wild ride down past all the stores on the main drag, until the course made a sharp left and then veered right about halfway down the next hill that took us out of town. Eventually it looped around, and we arrived back at the racetrack from the opposite direction. The stands were full of spectators, so it was a nice way to finish. I received a cool plaque for my efforts, finishing in 33:34 and I promised I'd be back the next year.

A couple of weeks before the '83 Canadian Games for the Disabled, Variety Village hosted the 2nd Annual Track and Field Classic at Birchmount Stadium in Scarborough.

This time the featured race was an Open Class 1500 metre that pitted a couple of America's best in Gary Kerr and George Murray, against a foursome of Dan Westley, Mel Fitzgerald, Rick Hansen and Andre Viger. Ron van Elswyk and I rounded out the 8-man field.

I knew I was in over my head against this group, but it was a great opportunity to test my fitness level against some of the best. Graham wanted me to go as hard as possible and stay as close to the field as I could. He made a point of telling me to give it everything I had, even if I came last. If I make the effort, I might be rewarded with a personal best.

It was super fast and when the race was over, Dan had nipped Gary at the wire, winning in the world record time of 3:57.70 vs 3:58.09. Mel stopped the clock in 3:58.30, Andre in 3:59.10, Rick in 3:59.20 and George in 3:59.40. I indeed set a personal best of 4:22.7 in finishing seventh.

I was amazed that Gary was so close to Dan's time. This was a perfect example of how the positioning of the knees negated much of the effect that the abdominal muscles played in the transference of power from the arms into the chair. Years ago, the mention of a Class 2 athlete giving a Class 5 racer a run for his money, would have gotten you laughed at.

This competition impacted the sport of wheelchair racing in another big way, since news of the event reached far and wide. The International Paralympic Committee sent their congratulations to Variety Village, and Variety's Paul Gains was contacted by the Los Angeles Olympic Committee organizers. They were contemplating holding an exhibition 1500 metre wheelchair race in the 1984 LA Olympic Games.

Through the efforts of many individuals, the '84 Olympics did indeed include an exhibition 1500 metre wheelchair race. All thanks to the forward-thinking crew at Variety.

I knew going into the Sudbury Nationals that I would have to make a good showing to get on the Shadow Team for next year's Paralympic Games set for Illinois and winning the slalom title again after a no-fault run helped my cause, but my track results were not what I wanted. I felt my fitness level was good, but the wind and constant rain during the week didn't help much. The price I paid for being so light.

By the end of the competition, I had collected a handful of silver and bronze medals, but I was not convinced that my haul this time around would be good enough. I would have to sit and wait for the verdict.

At the end of September, Mel outsprinted Rick to win the Montreal Marathon by the slimmest of margins (1:59:10.78 vs 1:59:10.92). Ten days before this race occurred, the great Belgian racer, Gregor Golombeck set a new world wheelchair marathon record of 1:55:13 in Europe. All around the world, at all distances we wheeled, record times continued to fall.

We also got word that because of all the work put in by numerous individuals and organizations around the world, the '84 Paralympics would now include the marathon for the first time as a medal event. Another big step forward in our history.

By this time not having a job was starting to be an issue. My Unemployment Insurance was about to run out and that meant I would have to apply for a disability pension again. After having good jobs in the past, I was not keen on sitting at home. And if I wanted to continue to race, I would need a source of income.

Chapter 13: A Job for Life

One day in October, Bob Ellery and Marv heard about job openings at the War Amputations of Canada on Merton Street in Toronto, about a twenty-minute drive from where we lived on the Esplanade. The two of them went up there and after talking to the Supervisor, they were hired, along with Brien.

Their job was making the metal key tags that the War Amps sent out to Canadians, tags that if you put them on a set of keys and lost them for whatever reason, anyone who found them could drop them in the mail, and War Amps would do their best to see them returned to their rightful owner.

The other job entailed stuffing address labels into envelopes, which contained information about their services to the war veterans, and the programs initiated to help child amputees.

The thought of stuffing envelopes for a living did not appeal to me in the slightest. It seemed demeaning and after working for the Bell in a few meaningful capacities, I thought this was a step backwards.

After a couple of weeks, it seemed that the guys enjoyed working there though, not to mention they were getting a steady paycheck. Not a lot, mind you. No-one works for a charitable organization of any kind and expects to get rich.

But about three weeks after the guys had started working there, John Klis and I found ourselves in line on a dingy street downtown, waiting to pick up our cheques with the rest of the people in need. At some point we looked at each other and decided once was enough. Back home we asked one of the guys to talk to the War Amp's plant Supervisor once more, and within a week John and I were War Amps newest employees.

Not long into the job I realized it was nowhere near what I thought it would be. It was all in your perspective. The tasks we did back then certainly didn't need the brains or the skill of a rocket scientist, but it wasn't hard to see the good that the organization did, and to understand the magnitude of assistance that the War Amps provided by distributing these address labels and the key tags.

Especially the key tags. The War Amps have returned literally hundreds of thousands of sets of keys to people all over the world and their letters of gratitude were heart-warming. Some were keys they needed immediately, and some were keys that were irreplaceable for sentimental reasons.

Just as important, War Amps provided work for dozens of veterans, all disabled during combat in various degrees, with work. The vets were the driving force that made the metal key tags and address labels. Back then there were no computerized machines to help make the job easier and faster. Just old machines that barely did their job without the constant maintenance required to keep them up and running.

They would tell us tales of life in the Army, or the Air Force or the Navy. No matter what happened to them, the injuries were the price they were willing to pay for our freedom. Some stories would raise the hair on the back of your neck, all told in a matter-of-fact manner.

But that was the way it was. Things had to be done. Period. Regardless of the cost. And while they worked out of a sense of duty, we made up games to keep our minds engaged. Who could cut the most labels in a day? Who could stuff more envelopes? We had quotas of course, but we managed to get stuff done while still having a good time.

Some of us worked there for more than two decades, and we were overjoyed when we moved into the new building in Scarborough. It was a longer drive to work and back, but new machines and the new programs that were initiated kept us going. Marv became a supervisor, and I became the Health & Safety Officer. Eventually I became the Video Co-Ordinator for the vast collection of war films and the many videos that War Amps made that chronicled the success stories of the many disabled children who's prosthetics were supplied by the Organization.

Staying almost thirty years at one company was bittersweet though. The nature of my fellow employees was such that many died early, due to their injuries and it was always painful when someone who had given up one way of life to go to war and come back forced to take another of life's paths, only to see them die before their time, seemed so unfair.

By the time I retired in 2010, almost all the veterans were gone, as well as many others, including my long-time teammate and great friend John Klis.

I played ball with the Spitfires for a couple of seasons, but over the summer there was enough interest in building another team from scratch to play

Chapter 13: A Job for Life

in the Lake Ontario Conference, and so the Toronto Outlaws took to the hardwood for the '83/84 season.

Our first roster consisted of Brien Foran, John Klis, Randy Critch, Dale Moe, Marv Murray, Dennis Kloppenburg and me. We took our colours from the NFL Oakland Raiders and wore black and silver uniforms.

We didn't have a winning record that first year, but I was fortunate enough to win the scoring title in my Class, as well as making the Conference All-Star team, and while we only won a couple of games, we hoped to find more sponsors before the next season rolled around.

Chapter 14:
Silver Lining

By now, the sport of racing marathons had increased in popularity, with many athletes from many countries competing on road courses around the world. Almost all of the next wave of innovations to our racing chairs were a direct result of trying to overcome the obstacles that racing on the road presented, as opposed to wheeling on a smooth flat track.

On the track, the ability to turn corners without losing speed was our only obstacle, while out on the road, there were grates to contend with, holes in the pavement to go around, hills to climb, and sections of downhill where you could reach speeds that would make your front wheels chatter like a tree full of squirrels. Everyone wanted to go fast, but we wanted to be able to do it as safely as possible, regardless of international rules.

Bev and I had been going together for a few years and I no longer held that deep rooted fear of being abandoned, so when Valentine's Day rolled around in February, I decided to do something out of the ordinary. Never been much for Valentine's Day for decades and usually I got in the habit of giving a card to whomever I was dating at the time. That year I suggested dinner at a place on the Esplanade where we had gone before.

During dinner I mentioned that I had read in the newspaper that a Canadian destroyer was moored down on the waterfront, and I said before we head home, I'd like to check it out first.

She agreed and off we went. Only took ten minutes to drive there and while we sat in the parking lot, I gave her my usual Valentine's card, but with a poem I wrote inside. It took the third reading before the last line of

Chapter 14: Silver Lining

"Will You Marry Me?" finally sunk in and I got the answer I was looking for. 2022 will be anniversary number thirty-seven. Who says dreams don't come true?

In March of '84, I was voted one of 150 "People of the City" by Toronto Life magazine in celebration of Toronto's 150th Anniversary and I was invited to a fantastic banquet for everyone to meet one another and to hear each other's stories. It was quite an honour.

The March 1984 TORONTO LIFE magazine cover story was about 150 Portraits of the most influential, powerful, glamorous, opinionated, useful and creative people of the city. I was voted as one of the 150 but not sure what category I fit into! No doubt a good word had been uttered by their Editor Marc De Villiers. When he was a young student at Ryerson, he wrote an article about me for the Globe and Mail's Weekend Magazine, leading up to the '76 Games.

Toronto hosted the Ontario Games in June, and I had no problem winning my races, including the slalom. As well, I raced the Variety Village 10K Provincial Championships and came in 4th. A good number of out-of-town racers were now training at Variety Village in preparation for the Paralympics later in the year, and Newfoundland's Mel Fitzgerald obliterated my record from last year, winning in 29:24.

Just before the Lindsay 10K rolled around again, Variety hosted their 3rd Integrated Track & Field Classic at Birchmount Stadium. The featured event was an Open Class, 1500 metre race of invited athletes from around the world, here to put on a demonstration before the '84 Paralympics in Illinois, slated for the following month.

Most of our top Canadian racers were training elsewhere, but nevertheless, the race was unbelievably fast, with Belgium's Paul van Winkle crossing in 3:48.1 for a new world record. American George Murray was second in 3:48.5, Peter Trotter of Australia, third in 3:48.7, and Andre Viger of Quebec was fourth in 3:48.9.

Not sure exactly when, but word came down that a problem had arisen regarding the funding of the Illinois Paralympics and emergency measures dictated that the Games be moved to England. A funding crisis had forced a change in plans at the last minute and no other venue could be found in time. Stoke Mandeville would host the wheelchair and amputee athletes, while the blind and cerebral palsied competitors would now be competing in New York.

Over the years I have heard more than one reason for the sudden change in venue, but from a personal standpoint, I was happy to go to England regardless of the reason why. Stoke was the birthplace of wheelchair sports and England was my mom's home country, having moved here after WW2 as a war bride. Nothing against the USA, the Games would have been just as much fun and well run, but America was just down the block. I had plenty of time to race south of the border.

Fortunately, my sponsor, Speedy Muffler King, stepped into the breach and helped to fund the Canadian team, since expenses to send us overseas instead of down to the States, were beyond what had been allocated for the event.

Over in England, our men's track coaches were Tim Frick and Graham Ward, and the women were coached by Rosanna Ward, Heather Snell and Cathy Walsh. Our basketball coaches were Joanne Skillen and Spitfire's Bob Bryce.

The first thing a lot of athletes had to do upon reaching England was to start removing any equipment that was still banned by the Stoke rules. That meant no steering devices and the chair still had to have four wheels.

However, my teammate Paul Clark arrived in England intent on racing in the 3-wheeler that he brought from Canada. And when it was deemed illegal, he attached a matching front wheel that barely contacted the surface, but was good enough to pass inspection.

Luckily, I was still riding in the 'Rail', and I passed without any issues.

The official results, when the games were over, showed that the Canadian men's team brought home the most track hardware of all the countries, as seven athletes took home 21 medals during the days of competition.

While the Canadian paras were collecting their hardware, the quad division was dominated by Class 1B Jan-Owe Mattsson of Sweden. His revolutionary way of pushing his chair using a backhanded stroke technique would soon be adopted by quad racers around the world.

Previously, all classes used the "grab-the-rim, push-and-let-go" motion to propel their chairs. But one glaring difference for quad racers was the fact that they had varying degrees of lost strength and mobility in their hands, making gripping the hand-rim difficult if not impossible.

By using the back of his hands, Mattsson was able to exert more power to the hand-rims and therefore went faster, much faster. He added extra padding to the back of his racing gloves to protect them from the pressure and the rest was history. Before long this became the recognized way for quads to push their racing chairs throughout the racing world.

He got the idea from a fellow teammate, who had broken his wrist but wanted to continue to train while it healed. When his friend went faster than he had ever gone before, Jan-Owe decided to try the technique on both hands and had great success.

The technique would see this class of racers go faster than ever before. During the time when quadriplegics were not allowed to wheel the longer track races, the Mattsson style of pushing, combined with the continued development of the racing chair, would allow quads to one day break the 2-hour marathon mark.

At the Paralympics in England that year, the future racing legend took home two track gold, winning the 400 and 800 while still having enough left in the tank to win the Class 1B marathon at the end of the competition.

In Class 2, Canada's Paul Clark won 5 medals on the track, winning the 800-metre gold and taking home the silver in the 200 - 400 - 1,500 and 5,000.

The only wheeler to beat him was the great Hans Frei of Switzerland. The Swiss racer won gold in the 1,500 and 5,000 and collected silver in the 800, bronze in the 200 and 400. The two of them would continue their battle out on the road when the marathon was held on the last day of competition, with Paul taking home the silver medal.

Australia's Mike Nugent won the Class 2 400 and bronze in the 800 and 1500.

The Class 3 sprints, the 100, 200 and 400 were a battle between a pair of Belgian racers and an athlete from West Germany. Marc de Vos of Belgium and his teammate, Paul van Winkle went head-to-head in all three contests. De Vos took gold in the 100 and 200 with van Winkle close behind, but Marc had to settle for silver against his countryman in the 400 final. Gregor Golombeck of Germany won the 3 bronze medals.

Canada's Andre Viger was content to let others contest the sprints since his focus, like a lot of the team, was on the marathon. He began his competition by wheeling to a bronze in the 1500, the gold going to van Winkle and the silver medal to Golombeck.

Gregor rebounded in the 5,000, holding off American's George Murray and John Rodolph for the gold, and his 5th of the Games.

Class 4 was dominated by Canada's Ron Minor. Over the years, with help from Graham, Ron had polished his pushing stroke to utilize his tremendous arm power and while he won the bronze in the 100, he struck gold in the 200, 400 and 800. He won the 200 over Remi van Ophem of Belgium and America's Randy Snow, the 400 over Snow and Australia's Peter Trotter and in the 800 over Trotter and Snow once more. Then he relaxed, in preparation for the marathon.

Fellow Canadian Rick Hansen lined up for the 1500 and held off Trotter and Snow to win the Class 4 final, but in the 5,000 it was Trotter who collected the gold. Rick settled for the silver, ahead of Jean Francois Poitevin of France. Like Mel, Andre and Ron, Rick's focus was on the marathon, and I think any medals he won on the track were an extra bonus.

Class 5 was the domain of Switzerland's Franz Nietlispach, who ran the table and won 5 gold, from the 100 to the 1500. Americans Dean Barrett and Tom Foran took home silver and bronze respectively, in the 100 - 200 and the 400 finals.

In the 800, Nietlispach was challenged by Australia's Robert McIntyre but still collected gold.

In the 1500 Class 5 final, Canada's Mel Fitzgerald entered his first race and picked up a silver behind the Swiss racer, with McIntyre taking home the bronze.

With Nietlispach on the sidelines, American Tom Foran won the 5,000 gold, Fitzgerald the silver and McIntyre the bronze.

Our quad relay team brought home gold in the 4 x 100-metre relay, while in the para relays, the foursome of Paul Clark, Mel Fitzgerald, Rick Hansen, and Ron Minor won silver in both the 4 x 200 and the 4 x 400. The Belgian team took gold at all 3 distances.

I would be doing a great disservice to the women if I left out the tremendous job they did on the track as well. If the guys deserved a "good job-well

Chapter 14: Silver Lining

done, then the ladies deserved a "great job-well done". Seven ladies won 22 medals, 17 of which were gold.

Ontario's Class 1A Martha Gustafson won gold in the 100 - 200 - 400 and 800 races and threw in a discus gold medal for good measure.

Class 1C Tham Simpson captured gold in all the same races as Martha and won the slalom as well. Class 1C Judy Zelman took home bronze in the 200 and 400.

Class 3 Debbie Kostelyk of Alberta collected gold in the 100 and 400 and a silver in the 200. BC's Diane Rakiecki brought home a silver from the Class 4 800 final.

Angela Ieretti of Ontario won gold in the 800 and 1500 and 5,000 metre races and a silver in the 200 and 400, in her Class 5 events.

The women won gold in their 4 x 100-metre relay to cap off a successful competition.

I went as fast as I could in my 100 and 400 races but ended up out of the medals. What bothered me the most was the change in barometric pressure that I felt when we arrived overseas that triggered my propensity for getting migraines.

On a bad day at home, I can be found in my room, in the dark, trying not to move a muscle. Most times chewing a few nasty tasting pills and chilling out for a few hours did the trick. In England, it just remained a dull throb throughout the week.

I never felt right, but it didn't contribute to finishing times that kept me out of the medals though. These things happen, and with the depth of the assembled competition, there were certainly no guarantees that even with a clear head, I would have had enough speed to reach the podium. Regardless of circumstances, the outcome is the bottom line.

Since I failed to medal in my sprint races, it again fell to the slalom to be my ticket to the podium. This time around the course was laid out on the backstretch, although we wheeled the race in the opposite direction. As usual, the competitors in each class pulled a number from a hat to decide the start order. Unfortunately, American Dave Williamson was absent from these Games, so we had no opportunity to break our personal tie of one gold each.

But my slalom chair was something that got a lot of attention. I had the frame spray-painted red, my new upholstery was red and my 20" knobby red tires without hand-rims opened a lot of eyes as we gathered around the course before the race began.

There were well over a dozen competitors in my Class that put their hands in the hat, but I pulled out # 1. That got my adrenalin pumping right away as I began to take another quick look at the layout before I was called to the start line. I like going first to put pressure on the field, but it only works if you put down a clean run. Penalty points usually spell disaster.

One thing I had noticed was that the straightaway portion was rather short. Maybe not even long enough to hit top speed. But there were a lot of gates around the ramp and jump platform, plus having to duck under a half dozen bars suspended overhead that were part of the final straight. I decided to let a bit of air out of my tires.

I had a great run. The softer tires did make for better turns on the track surface, and I incurred no penalty points as I raced to the finish line. I was low enough on my 20" tires that I barely had to duck to get under the final obstacle on the way to the finish line.

Then it was a matter of waiting as each athlete took their turn. It was nerve-wracking I can tell you that. As each athlete failed to beat my time, I got more and more excited.

Eventually enough racers had completed the run that I realized I had the bronze in my pocket. Then there were two competitors to go, and then just one. Osawa of Japan was the only competitor left, and I guess the best was saved for last. The Japanese athlete raced through the course, penalty-free and beat me by 2/10th of a second. Ouch! Belgian's Paul van Winkel won the bronze.

So close, and yet so far! I could almost taste it, but I was more than happy to win the silver medal. It was one up from the slalom bronze I won 8 years before in Toronto, and more importantly, I added to the team's total, and I didn't go home empty-handed.

While the medal haul among the Canadian racing team was impressive, the real objective had yet to be realized. While American racers are credited with completing the first wheelchair marathons in history, over

Chapter 14: Silver Lining

the years Canada had also become a strong voice in the movement to push for the marathon to be included in the world championships and the Paralympics going forward.

Once we knew that the marathon was going to be contested for the first time, that became the main objective for some of our racers. We had come a long way from racing old rickety wheelchairs down the hospital halls in decades past. It was time to hit the road.

Our marathon team was comprised of Mel Fitzgerald, Rick Hansen, Andre Viger, Ron Minor, John Boyko, Paul Clark, Serge Frechette, Ross Sampson, Lenny Marriott and me. Our medical team of Dr. Michael Riding and Dr. Emilie Newell were present at our spaghetti-loading dinner, to offer up advice and to make sure we had no underlying issues. We were excited and ready to roll.

As planned, at the gun, Rick, Mel and Andre sprinted out in the lead, with the rest of the world in hot pursuit. Their plan was to work together, and create a gap, with the intent of leaving the rest of the field behind. I found my own group to work with and went out hard.

At the tape, Rick and Mel were side by side, and Rick rolled over the line first and into Stoke Mandeville history, winning in 1:49:53. Mel's time was 1:49:54. Andre was not far behind and when everyone had crossed the line, Rick had won the Class 4 gold, Mel had the Class 5 gold, and Andre had the Class 3 gold, crossing the line in 1:54:41. Paul Clark won the Class 2 silver and Ron Minor won the Class 4 bronze.

I felt good on the road, pushed hard and finished strong with a personal best time. I came short of the Class 3 podium though, rolling through the line in 2:19:42, and good for sixth place. Top 10 in my Class? I'll take it.

Paul was beaten for the Class 2 marathon gold by Switzerland's Hans Frei, with Graham Condon of New Zealand winning the bronze. When Andre won gold over Gregor Golombeck of Germany, Canada's Ross Sampson wheeled home for the bronze. Sandwiched between Rick and Ron Minor, Jean-Francois Poitevin of France took silver in the Class 4 race and Americans Brad Hendricks and Tom Foran won silver and bronze behind Mel Fitzgerald in Class 5.

Coming home with a Paralympic silver in the slalom (54.84) and a good showing in the marathon, helped mask the disappointment of not getting a medal on the track. And from looking at all the machines that raced on the track over the week, I knew I had to modify my chair once I got back home to Canada.

Later in the year, the LA Olympics did indeed feature an exhibition 1500 metre wheelchair race. On August 11, 1984, after a series of separate races around the world, the 8 fastest wheelers at this distance assembled at the LA Memorial Coliseum and in front of 70,000 spectators put on a race that is still talked about and watched on YouTube to this day.

Rick, Mel and Andre represented Canada in that international field of world class racers, with Americans Randy Snow and Jim Martinson, Belgian Paul van Winkle, Peter Trotter of Australia and Jeurgen Geider of France rounding out the field.

Going into the race, it was all about the best strategy, for it could play a major role in the outcome. No-one wanted to lead the pack and have the field draft off them, only to have a racer pass them near the end. And no-one wanted to stay so close together as to have a crash during the event either. That was the last thing anyone wanted to happen while we were trying to show the world the excitement of wheelchair racing. But in the end, you had to be close enough to make it a sprint to the finish for a chance at glory.

It became a moot point when van Winkle sprinted away at the gun from out in lane eight and built a big lead while the rest of the field sorted out their initial wheeling order and formed a line ten chair lengths behind him. Meanwhile Paul continued to sprint, making no attempt to pace himself and continued to widen the gap between himself and the line of racers strung out behind him.

On the first lap, Jim Martinson of the US tried in vain to wheel van Winkle in, but he was unable to gain enough ground before he faded somewhat, and the pack caught up to him. As the race wore on, van Winkle continued to lead, stretching it out even farther at one point.

On the last lap, when his pace was finally beginning to slow, there still was no-one willing to make a run at him, so he led from start to finish and left the rest of the field to fight it out for silver and bronze. Winning time: 3:58.58. And he did it all alone with no help from the rest of the field. It was a dominating performance. The rest of the racers spread out once they reached the straightaway, and then it became a sprint to the finish line. American Randy Snow took silver and Canada's Andre Viger won bronze.

Back home, I wheeled a few road races and finished the season by winning the Miller Light Life Toronto Marathon in late September against a couple of local racers. There were still numerous sets of streetcar tracks to contend with and rough patches of road to wheel on, which contributed to my slow winning time of 2:38:18.

And again, the basketball season left a lot to be desired. Though I made the Conference All-Star team once more, we didn't have a lot to show for in the standings. Only two wins again were not what I had hoped for. Trying to coach your buddies and play your game at the same time was proving more difficult than I had expected.

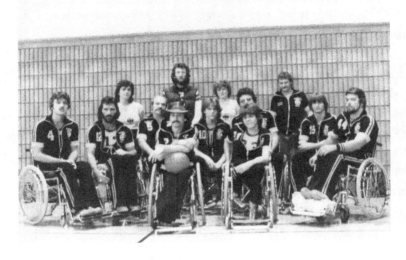

NWBA Scarborough Hawks team roster (l-r) (back row) Bev Waddell – Coach Gord Allen – Jacquie Phillips – Jamie Wasyluk (middle row) Stan Mason – Marv Murray – Dale Moe – Dennis Kloppenburg – John Klis – Don Alley – Brian Halliday (front row) Chris Stoddart – Tim Haslam

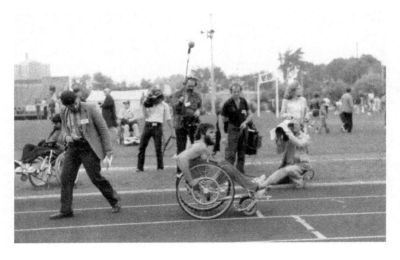

Bill Brouse warming up in our new SBS chair at the 1981 Scarborough Nationals, under the watchful eye of a Rules Committee official

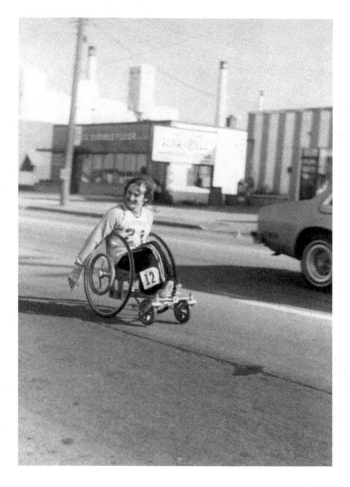

Wheeling along Lakeshore Blvd during the 1981 Toronto Marathon, becoming the first wheelchair athlete to complete the marathon

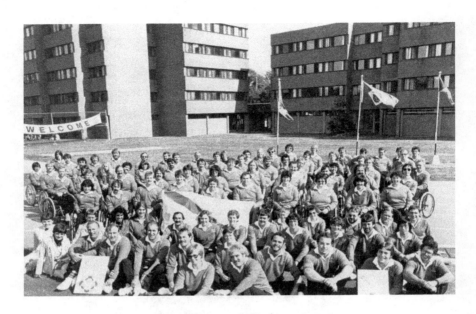

1982 Halifax Pan Am Games team photo

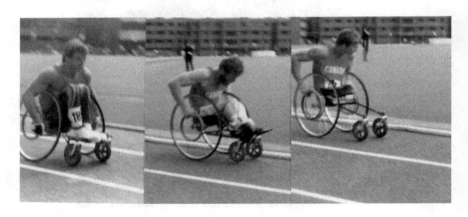

1982 Halifax: Rick Hansen – Mel Fitzgerald - Dan Westley

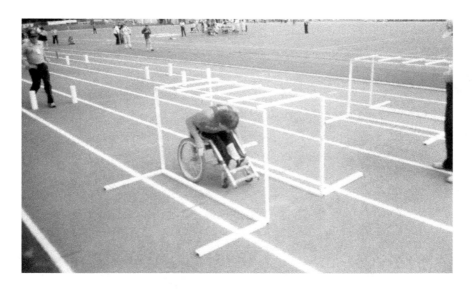

Winning gold in the Class 3 slalom final at the 1982 Halifax Pan Am Games

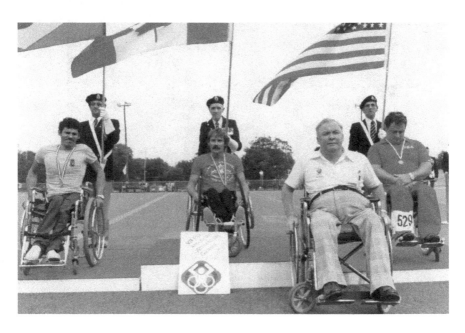

slalom medal presentation from Halifax, with American Dave Williamson winning silver and Juan Silva of Brazil the bronze medal

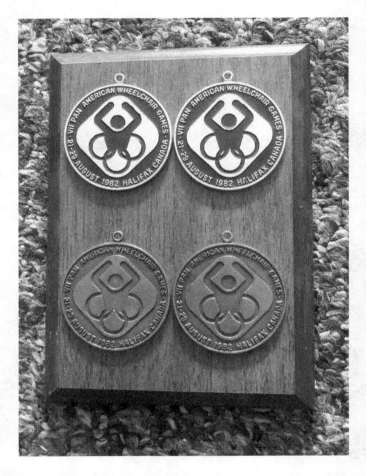

Halifax medals - gold in slalom and the 4 x 100 metre relay - bronze in the 200 and 1500 metres

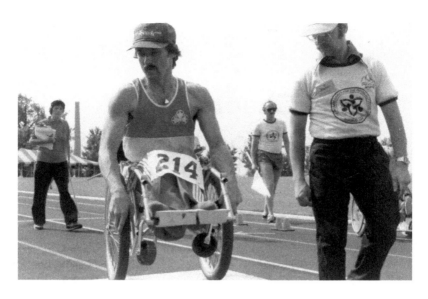

working through the slalom during the 1984 Ontario Games in Toronto under the scrutiny of wheelchair Hall of Fame official Barb Montemurro (far left)

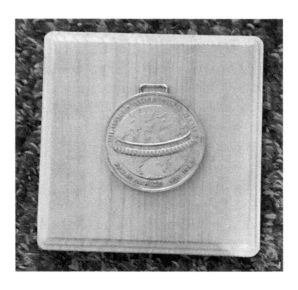

My silver medal from the slalom competition at the 1984 Paralympics at Stoke Mandeville England

Chapter 15:
A Year to Remember

1985 heralded in more world-wide advancements in wheelchair sports when Australia included wheelchair athletes in their National Games for the first time. They were held in late January and featured two invited international wheelchair racers, Paralympic gold medalists Paul van Winkel of Belgium and West German athlete Gregor Golombeck, who were flown in to compete against world-class racer Peter Trotter and his Australian teammates.

In Canada nothing compared to the announcement that wheelchair athlete Rick Hansen was planning to wheel around the world to raise money for spinal cord research and to raise awareness of the untapped potential of the disabled. There are numerous articles, books and souvenir programs that you can find if you want to understand everything that went on during the tour, but knowing he wheeled the equivalent of 3 marathons a day, for weeks on end, is mighty impressive. I'd be lucky to get out of Ontario.

He left Vancouver's Oakridge Centre on March 21st to begin the Man in Motion tour, and the first leg was one of the roughest as he wheeled down the west coast of America. As inspiring as he was to the thousands of well wishers that lined the road to cheer him on, donations were extremely limited.

He turned east from San Diego and headed towards Miami, but by the time he reached Texas, they had raised just $10,000 and they were wondering if the tour would be able to continue. But it did, and it was estimated that Rick pushed his chair 16 million times before the tour was over.

Chapter 15: A Year to Remember

The halfway point of the tour was in Melbourne Australia. Over 70,000 people packed Melbourne Stadium to wish him well.

Some countries went out of their way to ensure he had a trouble-free wheel through their country. Other places, not so much. In one country, a thief left behind all the valuables but stole Rick's complete training gear. In other countries, individuals vandalized his motorhome and teens in cars mocked and jeered as he passed through their town. But he continued regardless.

Rick was considered a hero in China, and had their full support, including being able to wheel up part of the Great Wall of China. He even received special permission to enter Russia.

However, for me, nothing was more important than the 25th of May, since it found me in St. Giles Church in Scarborough, getting married to Bev on her birthday. I was looking forward to beginning the best part of my life.

I did get bad news a month or so before the wedding when Graham informed me that he and his wife were going back to New Zealand. Since he was the National Team Head Coach in England the year before, I was taken by surprise. As usual politics played a role in his decision, and while I had other great coaches before I packed it in, it was Graham who helped me reach the top of the podium. The news was a blow that I had not expected because he was so much more than just a coach.

I was fortunate enough to be taken under another great coach's wing when Variety Village's Mari Ellery offered to help me out. Although I missed Graham, I learned a lot and wheeled some personal best while under her tutelage.

Back in the country from our honeymoon on Paradise Island in the Bahamas, I lined up for the Provincial Marathon Championships in Hamilton and came away with another hard-fought 2nd place for my efforts.

After the marathon was over, I took my chair to E & J for a little modification. I had them add a single mount in the centre. I knew that based on the all the different chairs that were used in England the year before, the 3-wheeler was going to be legal soon. It took less than a week, so I had plenty of time to wheel in the chair before my next competition date arrived. If it was deemed illegal come race day, I could easily put the pair of front wheels back on.

After wheeling the Lindsay 10K once more, I felt strong leading into the 4th Variety Village Integrated Track & Field Classic at Birchmount Stadium in Scarborough. A lot of the big names were absent from the competition, but the times were fast, nonetheless.

I got a good start in the 100 and held the lead the whole way until getting nipped at the wire by Spitfire's Dave Lash, who won in 17.34 to my 17.45.

The open 400 was a close race from start to finish, with the three medalists less than a second apart. Ron van Elswyk won in 1:10. I stopped the clock in 1:10.1 and Peter Trotter of Australia finished in 1:10.9 for third. The chair went around the corners as well as I expected and that had me looking forward to the upcoming National Championships.

In the featured 1500 showdown, Belgian Paul van Winkel set a blistering pace and left the field behind, winning easily in 4:11.55.

Our mid August Nationals in Sault Ste. Marie featured a lot of new names on the podium since many of the medal winners from 1984, had either retired, decided to take some time off, or in Rick's case, off wheeling on his Man in Motion Tour.

BC's Pat Harris ruled the sprints in my Class and Ross Sampson, who took the bronze in the '84 Paralympic marathon the year before, dominated the distance events. I settled for a silver and a couple of bronze, but I did keep my slalom crown with a no-fault run in the final.

Our relay team, consisting of veteran Ron Thompson, myself, Chris Daw and Dave Lash proved to be too powerful for the rest of the entries though, and we added to Ontario's medal total with a couple of gold in winning the 4 x 100 and 4 x 400 metre relays.

While my results on the track were not to my liking, I continued to lower my times out on the road. And out on the road, the racing chair was being transformed, as new equipment was developing rapidly. For a few years, it got to the point that you were looking at a new racer every year as more and more refinements were made and despite your best efforts, your new chair became obsolete seemingly overnight. I knew it was time for a new ride.

Chapter 15: A Year to Remember

Still running with 3 wheels, I entered a new wheelchair-only race called the Run for the Grapes 15K. It was set in St. Catherines and the course wound its way past the vast fields of grapes found throughout the countryside. It was a fun race, but it had a crazy ending.

Chris Daw bolted out into the lead, and I stayed with the pack. As we reached the finish line, we had one turn to make. All the spectators and an ice cream truck were stationed on the outside of the corner to cheer the athletes on to the finish line. Chris tried to navigate the corner at speed, but he ran out of room and crashed into the ice cream truck. I couldn't help but smile at him as he sat there watching the rest of us pass by on the way to the finish line.

At the end of September, I swapped out the single wheel and went back to my regular pair of front wheels to compete in the Miller High Life Toronto International Marathon once more. While the chair was stable enough on the track with the 3 wheels, it was kind of dangerous on the road. Since we now had our own Division, I was more than a little disappointed to be the only entrant, but I went as hard as I could and beat my personal best time from the marathon in England, breaking the tape in 2:18:0.

By now I was looking for marathons I could wheel in my area of Southern Ontario, but ever since I began wheeling marathons, I had heard how great the Detroit Free Press Marathon was for wheelchair athletes.

The wheelchair division was conceived through the extensive efforts of American quad racer John Boyd, and I heard it was a great experience. The race was set for a couple of weeks after Toronto, so I signed up.

It was a unique marathon in that it started in Windsor Ontario and finished in Detroit Michigan. And since it was so well run, it always attracted a big field of racers. It was as good as advertised and for years the Toronto/Detroit tandem of marathons were two races that I never missed if I could help it.

The race begins on the streets of Windsor and at the gun, it's a long sprint on smooth pavement to get yourself set for the tunnel that leads into Detroit. Flying down the Windsor/Detroit tunnel is quite exciting and for me, the best part of the marathon. And it's not too often that you start a race in one country and finish up in another.

The grade in the tunnel is steep, and you can really get rolling by the time you reach the bottom, and with other racers around you, there is not a lot of room for error. Last year's version of the Boston Marathon saw a huge crash on the slick road that injured more than one racer. With all the bad publicity that ensued, no-one wanted another pile-up so the negative people that wanted wheelchair marathons eliminated, had no further ammunition with which to used against us.

The fun of going down the tunnel is quickly gone as you begin to climb the circular grade that takes you back out into sunlight, and onto the streets of Detroit. Motor City roads were rough in many sections, but it was still fun to race with so many world-class marathoners.

To my surprise, I set a personal best time of 2:16:51, that was good for 3rd in my class and seventh overall. I realized there was a big difference in finishing times when you had to go it alone as compared to working with a group, and my reward was a beautiful pewter plate that was designed for this marathon, for finishing as Top Canadian.

In November, I got a call at work from wheelchair athlete Ron Thompson. Ron was a true pioneer in Canadian wheelchair sports, having competed for Canada since we first fielded a team in '67. At the time of the call, he was working for Variety Village, and had just gotten off the phone from talking with a gentleman from Barbados.

Variety Village was now known worldwide, and Carl Bayley, the managing director of the T. Geddes Grant Company in Barbados had called to say that they would like a couple of Canadian wheelchair athletes to compete in their Run Barbados Festival, which included a 10k road race on the Saturday, followed by a marathon the next day. Ron wanted to know if I would be interested in going to Barbados with him at the beginning of December.

Two races back-to-back are not something you would normally do, but a chance to be one of the first wheelchair athletes to compete in Barbados was too great an opportunity to turn down. Not to mention the all-expense trip to stay for a week at the Holiday Inn as guests of the Government of

Chapter 15: A Year to Remember

Barbados. War Amps gave me the green light and I gladly agreed. It was going to be an honour to wheel in these races.

The flight down was uneventful and once we cleared customs, there was a van waiting for us at Grantly Adams International Airport. We were met by Austin Sealy, the President of the local Amateur Athletic Association, and he drove the van to the Holiday Inn in Christchurch. We had a nice pool-level room and our hosts already had plans to show us the sights once the races were over. Things were looking good.

Mr. Sealy drove us around to show us the course layout so there would be no surprises on Saturday when we were scheduled to wheel the first of the two races, the 10K.

The race was a loop that started and finished at the beautiful Bay Street Esplanade, opposite the Prime Minister's office, and wound its way through Christchurch, along the historic Careenage, to the northern edge of Bridgetown. Then it continued through the main shopping streets and back to the Esplanade.

The 10K course began with roughly a 2 km uphill stretch of smooth pavement, before it turned left. After a km or so, the course veered left again, and began heading downhill through Bridgetown for another 3 km. This downhill section of road through the shops was made entirely of old cobblestones, laid down by hand literally hundreds of years ago. The cobblestones would make it rough to wheel over. We would have to be careful not to build up too much speed or we took the chance of losing control and crashing. Being much lighter, that was going to be a bigger concern for me than it was for Ron, who's added weight would be to his advantage.

At the bottom of the hill, the course turned left and back onto smooth pavement once more. In a Km or so, the course turned left again and from there it was a sprint up the incline to the start/finish line.

Since Ron and I were in different classes, it would have been possible for me to make a break right off the gun and pull away. However, we both agreed that these races were more promotional for us, even though they were sanctioned events. Our finish times were not that important, and considering there was just the two of us, racing alone would not be much fun and none too exciting for spectators. We agreed to stay together in both the races, and then have a final sprint to the finish. Best man wins.

Saturday arrived and the temperature was in the 90's. The race was set to go off around noon, as part of the overall Run Barbados festivities. The downtown harbour area was jammed packed with people, as they danced to the loud music that was blaring from huge speakers mounted on a large flatbed truck. Venders were everywhere. I have a great picture relaxing before the race, with a man's pet monkey climbing all over my chair and sitting on my shoulder. I love monkeys, who doesn't love monkeys?

Going into the race I felt relaxed. From a competitive standpoint, I was confident that I could cruise at Ron's speed and then use my 100-metre burst to overtake any lead he might have. At least that was the way I had it planned. Things can change though.

About two minutes before the start of the race, the heavens opened, and we got a full-fledged Caribbean sun shower that lasted all of five minutes. As if on cue, the rain stopped just before the gun went off. We were soaked and had no time to dry off, so with wet gloves and a slick pavement under our wheels, we made a rather slow climb up the road. By the time we reached the top and made the first left turn, I had a slight lead. The street had been lined with people since the beginning and everyone was cheering like mad as we wheeled past.

We had a good speed going on when we turned left again and began the descent through the main street of Bridgetown. Right away we were forced to control our speed. Being light was a big disadvantage here. The spaces between the cobblestones and / or their various heights, both threatened to flip me over. I had to slow down even more.

Meanwhile Ron had made up my modest lead, and while he also had to be careful about going too fast, his extra weight and the wider wheelbase of his chair was an advantage on this terrain. It enabled him to absorb a lot more of the bouncing around, the force of which was threatening to send me on a collision course with something hard and unyielding. Halfway down the hill he passed me and kept on widening the gap as we raced through town. People were everywhere. It was a sea of colours as people danced and waved as we flew down as fast as we could through the main street.

Up ahead I could see Ron beginning to turn left onto the good pavement, with about 300 metres on me when I hit the smooth section myself.

Chapter 15: A Year to Remember

He had a lot of speed built up as he began to push for the finish line, maybe 2 km away. I could still see him along the road in front of me as I made the turn, but in moments, he turned left again and vanished from view.

That was enough for me to put it into overdrive, since I couldn't remember exactly how far up the hill the finish line was, and I needed a bit of real estate if I was going to reel him in. I had good speed rounding the last corner and saw him up ahead of me.

His lead had shrunk since his momentum had dissipated and arm power was all that was left to get him to the end. Now he had to climb to the finish line and was slowing down. I picked it up right away and started to gain on him. The whole finish line area was teeming with people while the music continued to pound away. They were cheering loudly as I kept getting closer and closer. I managed to overtake him and finished in 31:00 to Ron's 32:11. Good racing.

Everyone was excited about how well the race went, and how fast we covered a course that was not ideally suited to wheeling at high speed. We sat and soaked up the festivities now that our work was done for the day. Plenty of water and lots of oranges to eat. People coming up and congratulating us and saying they were looking forward to watching the marathon the next day. Yes, the marathon...the next day. That should be fun.

The van took us back to the Holiday Inn and we basically chilled for the rest of the day. We knew that to beat most of the heat of the day tomorrow, the marathon would start at 6:00 am and the two of us were getting a half hour head-start before the field of runners would begin. That would be exciting. How long could we keep the runners at bay? Soon find out.

By the morning, based on the way the 10K unfolded, we had decided that trying to stay close to one another over such a long race was going to be difficult and we were going to get separated eventually. We decided not to wait for each other. The beginning miles were downhill, which would enable Ron to pull away and build a sizeable lead. There were stretches of cobblestone before we would reach smooth pavement at the bottom of this initial 10 to 12-Km downhill stretch, but not as rough as the main street of Bridgetown. Just like the 10K unfolded, I would have to try and reel him in once more. His lead would be a lot larger this time, and the last few kilometers or so, while smooth pavement, would be an uphill climb.

At that point in the marathon, I thought he might start to feel the miles and begin to pace himself to the finish line, which was situated at the Heywood's Resort, a government luxury hotel at the far end of the island. I hoped I would be in position to overtake him on the smooth pavement leading to the finish line.

Arriving at the Airport was a spectacle even more wild and crazy than the 10K race was the day before. Sunday, 5 in the morning and the Airport was rocking. A large group of runners limbered up along the beginning of the straightaway that led from the airport. A van was ready to follow us at a safe distance in case we ran into difficulties along the route.

At the gun, I was content to let Ron set the pace. I thought that if I could see him, I should be able to catch him if I timed it correctly. My power-to-weight ratio would only take me so far, and the longer a race went, the better chance a bigger man would have more left in the tank, but I had little choice.

The road was mostly regular asphalt, but like Bridgetown, the course did have stretches of cobblestone, mostly down the main street of the little towns we wheeled through. Eventually, we reached the old town of Oistins. Then the route took us along the south coast to Bridgetown, with a city dogleg to Eagle Hall. Then back to the city.

The middle part of the race seemed to go by in slow motion. It took less than a half hour once the race began, to feel the temperature rising as the sun made its way across the sky. Now it felt like someone was turning the island's thermostat up high. When I finally reached smooth pavement, I could see Ron in the distance. We knew the remaining miles would be smooth wheeling to the finish line, but also knew we had to wheel up the long hill to get there. The last chance for the course to task our arms and shoulders as we headed towards the end.

By this time, I decided I didn't want to play catch-up near the end. The way the heat was beginning to affect me, it made me realize I might not have a kick later in the race. Better to catch him now and stay at his pace and conserve energy for the finish. It took me a while to finally catch him and after a couple of miles pacing together, he told me to go if I wanted to, because he was going to have to back off his pace if he wanted to reach

Chapter 15: A Year to Remember

Heywood's in reasonable shape. Not surprising, considering we used up a lot of energy yesterday during the 10K.

With a feeling in my head that a migraine might be lurking in the future, I did pick up the pace. My reasoning being that I thought that the sooner I got there, the sooner I could take something for my head and then be able to lay down. I just had to continue along the Spring Garden Highway, along the west coast road through historic Holetown, to its finish at Haywood's, on the northern end of Speighstown. I was sure I could manage that.

Once I took the lead, the support van pulled up behind me and shadowed me for the rest of the race. With a couple of miles to go, I was running out of gas. The pavement was sizzling like a skillet. The heat waves coming off the road were as high as I was.

Then another problem arose. Rabbits... at first just a few would scamper across the road in front of me, but before long they were everywhere. Like lemming heading off a cliff, they just kept bounding out of the ditch on one side of the road and then disappearing into the tall grass on the other side.

This went on for maybe 400 metres or so, and it forced me to swerve back and forth across the road as I tried to work my way through. I thought for sure that if I ran one down, I would end up crashing. I made it past them, but by then, I could barely lift my head off my knees to see where I was wheeling. My head was on fire, and I felt sick to my stomach. Being forced to swerve all over the road had thrown off my equilibrium and I was dizzy. When I finally rolled through the finish line, I made a beeline for a section of grass and rolled to a stop.

I worked myself out of my chair and lay on the ground. I was done like toast. First-aid arrived not long after I hit the grass, and they began giving me liquids and a cold cloth for my head. I was quite content to relax in the shade of a big old tree, and wait for Ron to roll in. When he crossed the finish line not long after, and joined me in the shade, I asked him about the rabbits, but he saw none of them. They had all passed through before he got to that section. Lucky him.

Five or ten minutes later, Carl, and the crew in the support van came over to see how we were holding up. Carl said he thought I was going to crash on more than one occasion on that stretch near the finish line. I said I know.

It was like a moving landmine. Craziest thing to ever happen to me in a marathon for sure. Where the heck did all those rabbits come from anyway?

They looked at me like I fell out of the sky. There *were* no rabbits. I just suddenly started wheeling all over the road. They thought something had gone wrong with the chair at first. Then they had thought about pulling up beside me to see if I was all right, but I began wheeling straight again so they just continued to follow me.

They were just hallucinations? I really didn't believe them at first and quite frankly when it finally did sink in that there wasn't anything there, it did kind of scare me a bit. I would have bet the farm I saw hundreds of little brown rabbits hopping across the road.

My winning time was 2:36:06. Ron rolled through the line no more than a couple of minutes behind me. Peter Hermanns of Belgium won the main marathon in 2:28:46.

The post race festivities were held at the posh tennis courts in the resort. I was presented with a beautiful trophy from the Heywood's Resort for winning the 10K, and another award from the Government of Barbados for winning the marathon. All the hard work was done. Now we got to relax by the pool for the next few days before we had to board a flight back to Toronto. Variety would help keep me in shape as the winter months went by.

During the 85/86 basketball season we had more ball players than we ever had. Both Dale and Dennis came back to play, while Marv and Brien retired. We added rookie Shawna Petrie, my buddy Gino Vendetti joined, and we landed veteran Steven Little.

Steven was a veteran ball player and had suited up for the New Brunswick provincial team for many years. Not to mention we had raced against each other on the track and on the slalom courses countless times. He helped strengthen the team considerably, but it was not enough.

This was the last year for the Outlaws unfortunately, since things did not improve over the course of the season. Bev and I covered most of the expenses and while I did my best as player-coach, it proved too difficult to get everyone on the same page. As a result, we lost every game and not enough players were interested in playing another season.

Chapter 16:
A New Ride

I finally decided that I would buy another racer so I could take advantage of all the modern technology that the new chairs possessed. The biggest challenge was which company do I pick to build my chair? Seemed like every American racer worth their salt had started manufacturing their own version of a racing chair.

In the end I chose a chair made by Hand Crafted Metals in Florida. George Murray wheeled in it and the chair would be one of the many chairs that Rick used throughout his Man in Motion Tour. I hoped this chair would propel me to better times on the track and on the road. Time would show that on the road it was a good choice. On the track, not so much.

In terms of equipment, the small 8" front wheels and forks we had been using since the beginning of racing, were finally being phased out. They were being replaced by larger spoked front wheels, with rim diameters anywhere from 12" to 18", and they rode on high-pressure sew-up tires. Most chairs now came with a tie-rod system and custom front forks, much like the set-up on our 'SBS' chairs we built back in 1981.

Steering handles were now mounted on the new forks, attached in a position where you could reach them easily while in your tuck going downhill or while steering around corners or out of harm's way. The new front ends also came with an optional caliper brakes system like they have on racing bikes. Some races have steep hills, and you need something to slow yourself down. Most racers preferred to brake with their padded hands instead of a mechanical system though, because it eliminated weight and the chance of failure at an inappropriate time. Since there was a separate brake for each front wheel, you had to apply pressure evenly, or you were just as liable to skid out of control.

Another innovation on the new chairs was the invention of the road compensator. All roads slope towards the curb for water drainage, which meant when you wheeled on the road going with the flow of traffic, your right arm ended up doing considerably more work to prevent the chair from veering toward the ditch. These first compensators were usually a bar, situated within reach, that was attached to a mechanism that allowed you to turn the front wheels until you eliminated the incline. The wheels would stay in that position until you moved them back to neutral.

On the track the compensator soon became the perfect steering mechanism. On the road, you just kept tapping the bar until you were wheeling straight against the incline, but it didn't take long to realize that if you dialed in the corner on the track, it was easy to put something to block the compensator from moving any farther. Then you simply hit the bar as you went into the corner and again as you came out, to bring the wheel back to its original position.

However, the system had one large obstacle to overcome. It was deemed illegal for Stoke-sanctioned races, and it would be years before mechanical steering was permitted in the Paralympics.

With our rear wheel set-up now sporting custom hubs, bearings, rims and high-pressure tires, another big difference was how we now began to attach our hand-rims to the rear wheels. When we began racing, we had 24" rear wheels and 22" hand-rims, bolted to the rims with a spacer and a nut and bolt. When the 26" wheels and the smaller hand-rims made their appearance in Toronto in '76, these hand-rims had four or five L-shaped metal brackets that went out from the inside of the rim and then up to attach to the underside of the rear wheel rim. This added extra weight to the chair though.

Now we had a new set up. The hand-rims now had five or six small threaded tubes welded on them. The length depended upon how far you wanted your hand-rims away from the spokes. Next came the neat part. The metal screws that fit into the threaded tubes came with two round metal spacers. Each spacer had rubber on one side. The screws went

Chapter 16: A New Ride

through both spacers and the rubber sides were squeezed together onto the backside of the spokes.

Provided you made sure they were centred properly on the hand-rims, didn't wobble when you spun the wheel, and all the rubber spacers were pinching the spokes from behind, you were good to go. The best feature was that you could now have multiple diameter rims at your disposal and be able to switch them out in a matter of minutes once you got the hang of centering them properly. A lot of racers used smaller diameter hand-rims when they were competing in shorter distances, and larger ones for the longer races. You just had to remember to grab your tires for deceleration or you took the chance of pulling the hand-rims right off the wheels!

I was more than a little excited when my new HCM chair arrived from Florida in mid-February but looking at the frame, the measurements seemed incorrect. It seemed wider than I had expected, and on the track, my body was sliding to the right as I tried to make the corners at speed. Not to mention I had to extend my arms out farther to reach the hand-rims. I'd have to make modifications to rectify the situation.

My first opportunity to try the new chair on the road under race conditions, came in May when I once more entered the Ontario Wheelchair Marathon Championships, held in Ottawa this time, as part of the National Capital International Marathon. It was time to see how the new chair worked out on the road.

In an Open Class field of a dozen or so racers, Chris Daw and I worked together and left the pack behind. He put some distance between us as we climbed Parliament Hill and I couldn't close the gap on the flats through the last mile of the race. He finished in 2:24:20, I took second in 2:27:50. Hated being a bridesmaid again, but I still needed to solidify my sitting position.

Back home, my measuring tape told me exactly what was wrong. My rear wheels were mounted 2" wider on both sides when I compared it to my old frame. The pain I experienced in my arms was because I had to wheel with my elbows flared out to be able to reach the hand-rims. Fixing this problem was not going to be easy. Short of cutting the chair in half and welding it back together, I had to come up with a solution.

In June, after spending more than a year on the road, Rick Hansen began his wheel of eastern North America, leaving Miami in near 40-degree temperatures. He spoke to the top medical researchers at the National Institute of Health along the way, but he received no publicity and managed to raise just $20,000 on that segment of his trip. Not until he reached Canada did the hype, the enthusiasm and the funds begin to roll in.

Starting in Newfoundland, he began to have company as he wheeled across Canada. Retired racer and former teammate, Mel Fitzgerald was the first of many wheelers to keep him company as he ate up the miles. Back on the mainland, it was a steady stream of wheelies who rolled along for support. Athletes and non-athletes alike lined the streets of whatever town he wheeled through.

This became a common sight. Wherever he wheeled across Canada, area wheelchair athletes would be there to wheel with him. Many travelled to meet him at area rest stops. Sometimes for a mile or so, sometimes for days, Rick would find himself with company as he pushed through the final leg of his tour.

One day in mid-June while I was working in my office at War Amps, filling out paperwork, Bob Ellery called me into his office and wondered if I would be interested in jumping off the CN Tower on July 1st, Canada Day. Say what?

The TV show THRILL OF A LIFETIME was taping individuals whose "thrill" it was to rappel from the CN tower to the ground below, and Front-Line Rescue, a Brampton-based rescue consulting firm was raising money for the Peel Memorial Hospital by performing a mock high-altitude rescue to show off the sling the team had developed to get skiers off mountains when they had been injured. As an opportunity to highlight the capabilities of wheelchair athletes, we were asked if we would climb into the sling and go off the tower from above the restaurant.

The plan was to stretch a massive 2,300 metre nylon Dupont rope that would be wrapped around the CN Tower above the restaurant at one end, and long enough until it reached all the way to the Bathurst St bridge. This was before the Toronto SkyDome was built.

Was I into it? I sure was. This was right up my alley and might even rival the greatest stunt I ever pulled off back in high school.

Chapter 16: A New Ride

Our small town of Arthur had its own water tower with ARTHUR painted on both sides. One Halloween night, two of my buddies and I climbed the tower and using fluorescent orange paint, wrote "CONNIE WAS HERE" along the side of the tank in large letters. The gentleman in question was the town Reeve and he hated us long-haired rock and roll lovin' teenagers and we decided this was a good way of sticking it to him.

It was no easy feat by any means, especially for me. While my two buddies had no problem climbing up the ladder that was attached to one of the 200-foot tower supports, my legs got caught up in every rung as I pulled them up behind me. I realized that I would not make it up this way, and so I reached around and hung from the inside of the tower support. With the brush in my teeth, I just went hand over hand with my body hanging free of the support and I was up in no time.

Too short to actual do any painting, I sat on the metal walkway while they painted a large fluorescent orange ball on one side, wrote the message underneath and then we headed back down. I went down the same way I went up, and when we reached the bottom, the guys' said they were kind of freaked out watching me go down from the inside of the tower support. But I made it, no problem, and we made a pact to tell no-one of our stunt and to just let it ride.

At night, our work glowed like the sun, and on Monday it was the talk of the school, if not the town. Kids thought it was great, the adults were none too pleased, my dad included. Before school was out for the day, the OPP came by for a chat. There was no police force in Arthur and so the OPP held jurisdiction on any mayhem our little town might experience. Since no-one knew anything, or nothing was forthcoming, the matter became unresolved. The volunteer firemen went up the tower after a couple of weeks and painted a giant grey square where our note was. Case closed. Um, not quite.

After it was repainted, and thinking all was clear, a couple of un-named individuals began to take credit for the deed, and by word of mouth it reached the wrong ears. Before long someone came a-knocking and their parents had to cough up the cost of the paint to cover the slogan. No-one believed them when they said they were just kidding. The three of us kept that secret for a long time and the legend of the great Water Tower Caper was born.

Fast forward a decade and I was an invited guest at our school's sports banquet to talk about my career in wheelchair sports. After I had finished, I asked if there were any questions and the first thing they wanted to know was, was the story their parents told them about me climbing up the water tower true? It was, and now I had the chance to turn the "thrill notch" up to max and go off the CN Tower!

Bob and I met with all the crew, and they decided to make a trial run off the Hamilton Escarpment. We went out there and got all set to go but the day was windy, and the terrain was much more challenging and not to their liking. Once we showed them that we could get in the rig without much assistance, it was decided we were good to go.

Bev was not thrilled with the whole process. While she had no problem with me jumping off the tower if I wanted to, she was not looking forward to going up the tower herself so that she could bring me my chair once I landed down in the CN rail yard. It took a bit of convincing to get her to step out onto the roof of the restaurant. Back then, only a thick cable that stretched around the outer edge of the tower prevented anyone from falling over.

July 1st arrived, and Bob had the honor of going first. After getting strapped into the sling, they pushed him off the edge and then controlled his descent, so he smoothly rolled down the rope to the landing spot. Problem was, he didn't weigh enough to stretch that huge Dupont rope far enough, and at the lowest point of decent they had just managed to grab his feet and pull him down to the ground so they could get him out of the sling.

When it was my turn, they realized I was even lighter and that they wouldn't be able to reach me when I got to the bottom. One of the rescue crew said no problem. We would hook ourselves together and set a world record for the longest tandem traverse instead. Once clipped together, he jumped off, and took me with him!

Well, the rope stretched quite a bit and with both our weight we dropped a good twenty feet before we began to spring back. That got my heart pumping! Since he was a pro and an old hand at heights, he guided our descent manually so we stopped numerous times so that he could fish out his camera and take a few pictures while I gazed around speechless. We

Chapter 16: A New Ride

stopped outside the restaurant window and freaked out the people having lunch before continuing down the rope until we touched ground.

That night there was a big party in the CN Tower restaurant and a week later we watched the show on TV. What a great experience.

In mid-July I did wheel fast enough at the Ottawa Ontario Games to win my races, but the times were not up to par, and I wasn't all that surprised when three days later I got a call from CWSA to tell me I did not make the team going to Stoke, nor to the big track competition in Sweden later in the year.

I started to feel like the days of me winning a medal for Canada were numbered but took solace in the fact that perhaps I hadn't maxed out my personal bests yet. But somehow, I had to eliminate my butt from sliding out of position as I tried to take corners at speed. If I couldn't solve the problem, I would be hard pressed to put down times on the track that would make me competitive.

While the racing chairs continued to evolve and the times continued to drop, a French racer unveiled a revolutionary way of propelling his chair during the Kaiser Roll 10K road race down in the US during the summer. So much so, that racers from around the world would adopt this style, much like the quad racers copied the Mattsson technique to achieve personal bests.

Remember when you were a kid and used to turn your bicycles upside down and spin the wheel as fast as you could? And once it was going too fast to grab, you used your open hand to fan the wheel to make it go even faster? Jean Francois Poitevin of France began to use that technique to begin his races instead of the traditional grip-push-let-go style of wheeling.

By heavily padding his hands, he pounded down on his hand-rims that were mounted close to the spokes and continued that stroke for the duration of the race. He also wheeled with a distinct camber to his back wheels which helped in applying pressure to the hand-rims and helped to keep his hands from sliding off.

Poitevin finished the 10K in 24:34. with Canada's Andre Viger a close second. It was a window into the future. One day, every para racer in the world would use this technique as the world records continued to be lowered.

Since I wasn't headed to Stoke, I went out on the road and wheeled the 10K Lindsay Milk Run in July and joined a pack of local wheelers to compete in the Run for the Grapes 15K around St Catherines once more. Once done, I set my sights on the Toronto and Detroit Marathons.

The Toronto Marathon was on the last Sunday of September, and since I was the lone entrant again, I intended to take it out early and not stop until I ran out of gas. I was hoping for a personal best while still trying to figure out how to solve the problem of the chair's extra width.

So, at the gun, I took off down the road, and focused on getting into a steady rhythm that would take me to the finish line. At about the 5-mile mark, I had built up speed and was heading down the road at a good clip towards a major intersection. It was manned by one of Toronto's finest, who was holding traffic while the marathoners passed through.

Unfortunately, a little old lady did not heed, or did not see or hear the policeman yell a warning to her to not cross the road. She stepped off the curb and walked straight into my path. With no time to make a defensive manoeuvre, I grabbed my back wheels, closed my eyes and ducked my head.

We made quite a mess. While not a lot of blood was spilled, she took quite a tumble. Her purse blew up like a hand grenade and scattered the contents all over the intersection. I had to disengage what was left of her purse from one of the front forks before I could continue, with a flat tire and a rim that had a decided wobble to it. Luckily, I limped to the finish line and stopped the clock at 2:32:37, but even with the help of the new road compensator, my right shoulder ached for a couple of days.

A couple of weeks later, Bev and I drove to Windsor in preparation for the Free Press Marathon. The weather wasn't as chilly as the year before, so it was a comfortable race. I went out with the first pack at the gun, but they left me before we reached the tunnel, and I had to be satisfied with working with another group of wheelers who caught up to me.

In the end I won myself another cool pewter plate for coming 3rd in my Class. My finishing time of 2:19:11 was good enough for 7th overall. It was another great weekend, and I was happy with my result, though my shoulders

Chapter 16: A New Ride

ached, and my elbows were tender for more than a couple of days. On the road I didn't slide around in my chair as much as I did on a track but reaching over my wheels to grab my hand-rims was still a problem.

While not able to set a personal best time, I knew it was partially because I had wheeled the marathon using an old pair of rear wheels and a different diameter set of hand-rims since I had to send away for parts after the Toronto race. I was hoping to pick the new parts up in Florida since Bev and I had decided we were going to head to Miami in January, so that I could wheel in the famed Miami Orange Bowl Marathon.

In November, Gino and I joined a group of wheelchair athletes who wheeled with Rick, as he passed through Oshawa on his way to Variety Village in Scarborough during his Man-In-Motion tour. He received a hero's welcome when he reached Toronto, with a dozen of us tagging along for support.

After a few days rest, many interviews and press conferences, Rick once again led more than a dozen of us from Queen's Park Circle in Toronto along the QEW highway to the Ford Plant in Oakville before he continued west alone.

Eventually he reached Vancouver to another hero's welcome as the tour was finally completed. The impossible had been achieved.

The downside to this was that his racing career was finished. It would take months for him to recover from the ordeal and his shoulders would never be the same. Considering how dominant he was on the marathon circuit and on the track when he embarked on the tour, I have no doubt he left many gold medals on the table for others to win in his absence.

In December, Ron Thompson and I were again invited back to wheel in the Run Barbados Marathon. Ron still worked for Variety Village, but he did not do as many competitions, so he decided to send one of the athletes he was training, in his place.

Ron Robillard was a powerful marathoner and close to a dozen years my junior, so I had no visions of repeating as champion at either distance. He was determined to win, so I soon realized we would not be putting on a show like his coach and I did last year. Ron would go all out from the gun and not look back.

My aim going in, was to lower my time from the year before if I could, and to just let things play out. I would have to wheel my own race and hope for an opening. I knew from experience that a lot can happen in a marathon, considering its length.

Besides, I'd get to visit Barbados again and this time Bev would be coming along. We'd get a chance to relax by the pool and enjoy the sunshine at the Rostrevor Apartments where we were staying for the week.

No rain for the Saturday 10K, and there were tons of excitement and noise. The music was blaring, and everyone was dancing like all-get-out. Just like I remembered.

As expected, Ron bolted up the incline at the gun, and was a good 100 metres in front of me by the time I reached the top. Wheeling over the cobblestones through Bridgetown did not slow him down much, so I lost more ground on that downhill section.

Once he reached the good pavement, he ramped up his pace and had lengthened his lead by the time I wheeled off the cobblestones and onto the smooth road. I kept him in sight the whole race, but I didn't make much of an effort to close the gap. I decided to save some gas in the tank for the marathon. A five-thirty wake-up call comes early, and rabbits were on my mind. I went faster than the year before, so I was content with 2nd place.

Sunday morning came early and in no time, we were back at Grantly Adams Airport with the field itching to start the marathon. The omnipresent music was again pounding full bore from the back of the flatbed and the streets were filling up with people. They lined the course in all the towns we race through. Loved the excitement!

Hot and humid as per usual, so when the gun sounded, I let Ron take it out as quickly as he wanted. I decided to stay back at a comfortable pace and hope the heat might cook him a little bit. I would just have to wheel my own race, but still stay close enough to take advantage of anything that might arise during the duration of the marathon that might give me an opportunity to overtake him. Try as I might, I couldn't stay close enough, and he disappeared.

Chapter 16: A New Ride

So, I continued my steady pace and with about 5K to go, I saw him in the distance and realized he was slowing down. By the time I caught him, he was completely stopped. The seat frame of his chair had broken on one side, and he was rubbing against the moving wheel.

Bev was in the medical van that followed the leader, and they had pulled over to see if there was a medical problem. They were trying to help him as I wheeled past. Now was my chance. I had to put as much distance between us before he got it fixed and had a chance to run me down.

I managed to get a good lead but when I heard him coming from behind with about a kilometre to go, I knew it was not going to be enough. Having somehow bit through a coat hanger with his teeth, that Bev had found for him on the floor of the van (thank you very much), he had managed to tie his seat in place, and had just enough real estate to catch me before the finish line.

I gave it my best shot and reached my goal of posting a much faster time (2:32:00) and felt a whole lot better than I did the year before. No rabbits, thankfully.

While Ron won the marathon, he didn't get off without a scratch. During the race he had developed a huge blood blister that covered the whole palm of his right hand. Before Bev could see it and drain it properly with a pinprick to the edge of the blister, medical had taken him away and cut all the skin off the inside of his hand, leaving a giant open wound that bothered him for the rest of the trip.

I guess they were pleased with the results, since we were offered another week's stay at the resort. Unfortunately, Bev had to leave early, so she missed out on the trip that Carl and his wife Jill took Ron and I to on the far side of the island.

The beaches are amazing, but the undertow on that side of the island is treacherous and only the island's inhabitants know where it's safe to swim. The last stop, into the Harrison's Caves was also a unique experience, and a fine ending to another great experience in Barbados.

Chapter 17:
Reaching for The Top

As planned, Bev and I flew from Toronto via Air Canada to Miami in January where I intended to wheel the Miami Marathon, the unofficial World Marathon Championships. With wheelers from all over the world looking to get settled in their rooms, it took awhile before we unpacked and got to relax in the Eden Roc Hotel on Miami Beach.

As promised, the parts for my racer were there waiting for me, and I spent a couple of hours getting the chair ready for the marathon.

Race day was clear with a slight wind. It was hot, but nothing as oppressing as the heat I felt in Barbados. The race started and finished on the Island just off Biscayne Bay and it was cool to race across the Rickenbacker Causeway.

At the opening gun, I went out with the first pack of wheelers, but as the kms rolled by, more and more racers fell off the pace, me included. I found myself wheeling alone for a few kms, until I was caught by another group.

I stayed with this pack for the rest of the race and managed to outsprint most of them in the dash to the finish line.

My time of 2:16:14 was a personal best and put me 6th in my class and 18th overall. I was pleased. With Miami being one of the world's biggest marathons, finishing in the top 20 was more than I had hoped for.

The new parts worked fine, and the chair was one of the reasons I got a good time, regardless of its deficiencies, but after the race I couldn't help but check out a few of the race chairs that other guys were using.

One chair really caught my eye. American Marty Ball was wheeling in it, and he was one of the front runners during the race. This Top End racer had a hinged front end that was supposed to smooth out the rough section of the road. I might have to get me one of them.

Back home again, I raced on the indoor track at Variety Village, and in February headed down the highway to race in the Windsor Classic once more.

The Classic made its debut in 1982 and was an extremely well-run event. All the racers in this area made it a must-do competition. The facility had a 200-metre track, much like Variety, and its proximity to the northern US states meant there were always American athletes that crossed the border for a chance to race indoors during the dead of winter. Eventually the Windsor Indoor Classic would become the largest indoor competition for the disabled in North America.

The games were the brainchild of Celia Southward, who first joined the City of Windsor administration staff in 1976 as the Co-ordinator of Special Populations and Seniors. She was deeply involved in disabled sports throughout Ontario, and eventually, she would become both the President of the Cerebral Palsy Association and President of the Ontario Wheelchair Sports Association. Quite impressive in my opinion.

She always made sure the Classic lived up to its name, and all the decades of hard work and commitment made her 2011 induction into the Canadian Disability Hall of Fame a well-deserved achievement.

This year was the first time I raced at Windsor in the Master Class, instead of in my usual Class 3, so I took my 5 gold medals with a grain of salt. I did beat everyone in the 60-metre sprint, but stiffer competition in the longer distances resulted in me taking a backseat to better athletes, despite the colour of the hardware I took home.

I realized that the only way I was going to be faster was to be in peak shape and to do more work on the chair to stabilize my body. I could not afford to be moving around in the seat.

It was my own fault, but I realized when I first received the new chair from Florida that some of the dimensions were incorrect. Since the company was in Florida and I was in no position to go down there to get fitted, I had filled out the lengthy and complicated tech sheets and sent them all the dimensions that they required. Somewhere along the line there had been an error.

Now I was left with trying to add more padding around the inside of the cage to keep my hips moving from side to side and adding more camber to the rear wheels to get them as close as possible to the frame. Unfortunately, without a sponsor, I couldn't afford to buy another racer so soon.

A lot of the able-bodied road racers that I met while competing locally, rode bikes as part of their training, and like all athletes they wanted to ride on a quality machine. Many of the runners went to a bike shop near Yonge and Finch called LocalMotion. They had mentioned me to Leo, the owner, and he told them to send me to the store in case he could help.

Getting equipment for my chair sent up from Florida took time and cost considerably more money, once you factored in the shipping and the duty you had to pay. I was hoping I could find tires for both my back and front wheels without having them shipped from the US, and I wanted a place that I could take my chair to get the wheels serviced quickly.

I went to the store, and after telling Leo about wheelchair sports, he wondered if I'd like to be a member of his bike team. Members got a discount on equipment and repairs and there was a great long-sleeved Lycra racing shirt to wear during competitions. I eagerly agreed.

A few days later, I received a call from CWSA telling me I was in line to make the team going to Stoke for the World Championships later in the year and I made the shadow team for Korea in '88. There was a big racing meet in Sweden again and some of the top racers were headed there instead of going to England. There was an opening on the Stoke team. This was my opportunity.

Before heading out onto the road again, I entered another Variety Village Indoor meet. I always made it a point of racing at these meets if I could. I enjoyed racing here because I knew what it was like to grow up disabled and have no-one to aspire to. I knew I'd never be like my idol, Toronto goalie Johnny Bower, or any other athlete for that matter, but if wheelchair racing had been a sport when I was a kid, I would have jumped out of my stroller, maybe even my crib, to get in a chair and go racing.

I never considered myself too big of an athlete to enter any competition that would highlight the inner potential of disabled athletes. Plus, I liked to

Chapter 17: Reaching for The Top

go fast for the pure fun of it. Always have. I'm glad I did since I wheeled an 11 second 60-metre sprint for a personal best.

In May, I entered the Ontario Marathon Championships in Hamilton. Ron Robillard (Scanlon) led from start to finish, crossing the line in 2:08:06. I ended up second as usual, but as a bonus, the top two finishers got their way paid to Winnipeg for the National Marathon Championships in June. Excellent! Manitoba here we come.

The following month the Provincial 10K Championships were held at Variety Village. I rolled over the line in 3rd.

This year, for the first time, the track athletes that were being considered for National Team selection, went to a team fitness testing camp in Edmonton. For three days in the middle of May, we were put through a series of tests to determine our fitness levels and to pinpoint areas that required work.

The first test was to see how many laps an athlete could complete in 12 minutes. Easy enough. The next test used a computer to monitor each athlete as we wheeled a series of 60 metre sprints. That was kind of neat. I had never seen myself wheeling before.

For the third test, each athlete was videotaped wheeling on training rollers to produce a computer analyzed hand speed and technique video. CYBEX machine computations and body fat measurements of each athlete were included in the process.

The results, after everything was analyzed, put me in the middle of the pack for most of the tests and slightly higher in a couple of others. It was pointed out that one shoulder was stronger than the other and that needed extra work.

What was difficult to do was gain more weight as was encouraged by the training staff. I was still at least 20 pounds lighter than everyone else and the coaches wanted me to change my diet. But it's not something I hadn't tried before. I had been pumping weights at Variety at least once a week since the place opened and tried to switch my diet from chips and jellybeans to meat and potatoes, but it didn't help much. My best bench press in competition was 159 ¾ lbs, and that came after gaining a whole 5 lbs that took me to a whopping 95.

Thankfully my results at training camp were good enough to officially make the team going to Stoke in August. As well as entered in the slalom, I was advised to stick to the sprints and forget about the distance races. The way my chair continued to take corners, I was somewhat glad that I'd be going overseas as a sprinter, since being pencilled in to wheel the 100 and 400 metres, meant I only had to navigate a couple of turns per race. I could only hope the chair's poor cornering ability wouldn't affect the outcome of my races too badly.

Our national team was being sponsored by Adidas and I had the opportunity to go to their headquarters and pick out some new track clothes. While I was there, I was fortunate to meet famed sprinter Ben Johnson, who was getting a new wardrobe himself, in preparation for Korea. I was able to pick from a wide variety of clothes on a specific wall, while Ben checked out the whole room. When he realized I wasn't getting the opportunity to pick from all the same stuff, he pointed it out to the Adidas Representative, and he made sure I got to pick whatever I liked. Classy guy.

It was mid-June, the day before my birthday when I found myself in Winnipeg getting ready for the National Marathon Championships. It was a fast course, flat and smooth. Many racers set personal bests on this course and that's probably why the field was usually deep, with not only Canadian and American marathoners but with racers from around the world who travelled to Canada in search of a fast finishing time.

On race day there was a slight wind and moderate temperatures. Perfect marathon weather. Andre Viger led most of the way and broke the tape in 1:49:56 with Paul Clark second in 1:51:24. Ted Vince was a close third in 1:51:55.

I went out in a large pack, which included Australian Peter Trotter, American John Brewer, the great Jan-Owe Mattsson of Sweden and eventual women's winner, Angela Iereti of Ontario. I finished 9th overall, and 3rd in my class behind Andre and American legend George Murray.

Working in a pack enabled me to go faster than I had anticipated, and I set my all-time fastest marathon time, rolling over the line in 2:08:43. Making the Top Ten was an accomplishment I hadn't expected.

Chapter 17: Reaching for The Top

When July rolled around the '87 North York Ontario Games were next on the schedule. This was the 13th edition of the Ontario Games for the Disabled and much had changed since 1975.

There was lots of press leading up to these games because the Mayor of Toronto at that time was Mel Lastman and he wanted the event to be the greatest Ontario Championships ever. One of the reasons, no doubt, was the fact that they were expecting the then-Duke and Duchess of York to make an appearance.

The mayor's wife, Marilyn Lastman, worked tremendously hard and raised close to $400,000 in fund-raising events. I was quoted as being concerned that it might scare off other cities from hosting these events if the price tag was too high, but the mayor said I was being too negative.

Not everyone was looking forward to the Games, however. Former world cyclist Jocelyn Lovell had been rendered a quadriplegic four years earlier, after being struck by a vehicle while training, and he was quite against any form of disabled sports. He was quoted as saying he wasn't interested in "cripple sports" and he hated the media for portraying life in a wheelchair as fun. His involvement with Ray Wickson, then of the Spinal Cord Society of Canada, was one of the reasons the Society had initial problems with the Rick Hansen Man-In-Motion Tour. They felt all money should be funneled into research. It was successfully countered of course, since while everyone knew research was important, individuals had lives to live in the meantime and sports played an important role.

On the day before the games began, it was formally announced that the Duke and Duchess of York, Prince Andrew and Lady Fergie were going to officiate a men's and women's slalom demonstration in front of a packed grandstand during the Opening Ceremonies.

As reigning National Champion, I was to represent what training and hard work could accomplish, and sixteen-year-old Mubeen Jaffe would represent the future of our sport. We were going to perform in front of Royalty and that had my adrenalin going, for sure.

Leading up to the start of the event, they set up the slalom course on the track in front of the grandstand and by the time they had it completed, the stands were full of people waiting to see the Duke and Duchess.

Meanwhile, the photographers, who numbered in the dozens, were jockeying for position on the infield along the full length of the slalom course.

As I was getting ready to do my run, I was excited to get the opportunity to speak to the Duke and Duchess since the Duchess was going to start my race.

I have a great photo that my wife took right before the start. It shows me talking to Lady Fergie, but more important to me, is the fact that in the background I can see my late mother watching the proceedings with a big smile on her face. Time to do mama proud.

And I think I did. I had spent a lot of time perfecting my slalom chair, and hoped it was going to raise eyebrows in England later in the year. I flew through the course, never touched a gate, penalty-free... and then it was over in a flash. My national record set in Halifax had been 54.10. Now it was down to 53.45. I hoped I would be as smooth in England. Mubeen wheeled a good race as well, with no faults and that gave her confidence leading into the women's competition. This was just an exhibition after all, and the real slalom event would begin the next day.

During the weekend's races, I was being hard pressed by Kitchener's Ron Van Elswyk. Though I eventually won the slalom and the 100 metres to stretch my record to 15 consecutive wins at the provincials, I was second in three different distances to him during the competition. I was still unable to prevent myself from moving out of position when I hit the corners under a full head of steam, and I was fortunate to win Best Male Athlete of the Games.

Next stop Stoke Mandeville and the World Championships.

So excited to race at Stoke during the World Championships again, what with all its history. Not to mention the added excitement of having my relatives in the stands to watch me race.

The Games ran from late July until early August, and wouldn't you know, the slalom was the first event after the Opening Ceremonies, and it was unlike any slalom event I had ever entered.

To some, the slalom was the poor cousin to the "real races" and in the early days was often referred to as the "rehab event". Those of us who competed in the event didn't care. Try it yourself. See how easy it is. Anyone can go through gates but try doing it at full speed.

Chapter 17: Reaching for The Top

In the early days, you never knew what the slalom might entail. Sometimes they got quite complicated and sometimes a bit dangerous. Eventually it became a standardized course, though the obstacles themselves often changed order from competition to competition.

Perhaps to showcase the dexterity, speed and chair control the event was in fact highlighting, this year the event was a 2-day affair. One course on the Monday and a second different course on the Wednesday. That's an interesting development.

The first course was set up on the backstretch and in another twist, there were two parallel courses. Pairs of racers would go head-to-head in round one. Another first to ramp up the spectators, I guess. It's getting harder by the minute!

During my run I was lined up against a world class American road racer. This would be a challenge and it was. He was fast, just like I knew he would be, but he was too fast for his chair, for lack of a better word. He muscled his way through the gates and other obstacles but combined with the penalty points he incurred during his run; it ate up enough time to put him well back.

On the other hand, I had no problems. The 20" knobby tires had me stuck low to the ground, so there was no sliding as I manoeuvred around the pylons, and with no hand-rims, I had ample room on either side to attack the gates without fear of incurring a penalty. A third of the way through the course I knew he was not going to catch me. But how would my time stack up against the others?

Not to worry, at least not for the moment. My time of 51.5 had me leading the field by a couple of seconds, heading into Wednesday's finale.

The second course was indoors, and it was one large, complicated maze. So complicated that they gave each athlete a copy of the course to study, since they decided no-one would see the actual course until it was time to race. It was a lot to take in. The course was much longer and complicated than we were used to seeing. I knew what the consequences would be, if you got ahead of yourself, and lost concentration.

When it was my turn, I was ready to go, and at the gun I was off and working my way through the series of obstacles. The chair worked just like it was supposed to, and I was motoring my way along nicely. One complicated obstacle to go and then the finish line but as I wheeled my way through, I glanced up to align myself with the finish line, only to realize I'd be coming out of the manoeuvre on the wrong side of the last gate! Not again.

I hit the brakes and began to wheel backwards through the course, trying to retrace my exact route back to where I made the error. Part way back to the start of the manoeuvre, I realized where I had gone wrong. I corrected it and then went hell bent for leather through the maze again, out the right way and a final push over the finish line.

Even with all that extra work, it felt like a fast run. But it was agonizing to wait as each athlete took his turn trying to remember the correct sequence that would take them to the finish line as they raced against the clock.

After the dust had settled, and the times from both races had been combined, I had won the world slalom gold medal. I waited fifteen years for a chance to win at Stoke and it had finally come true. I was happy beyond words.

But, relaxing on my bed back in the residence an hour later, one of our team officials came in to tell me I had been bumped to silver once all my penalty points had been added up. He handed me my copy of the results and boy was I steamed. I looked at the printout of the course and where I accumulated penalty points. It was then I realized that they had given me penalties that I thought I didn't deserve. I went back to our team official and said I'd like to protest the results, since I thought I was unfairly given a 10 second penalty for something I didn't do. He shrugged his shoulders and said he'd go back to the officials and make a formal protest.

A couple of hours later, I was summoned to the official's tent to make my case. On the way, I met one of our team officials that was on the protest board, as she made her way to the tent. So, I explained my position to her on the way.

Usually, a slalom course is made up of a series of manoeuvres, each with a distinct entry and exit point. Even if you go back and redo the manoeuvre, once you exit the obstacle wrong, there is a 10 second penalty. However, on this course, the last obstacle was broken into two-parts, but on the printout, it clearly showed it was all considered to be one segment of the course. I said to her that I realized my error in the middle of the

Chapter 17: Reaching for The Top

obstacle, and BEFORE I made my exit, I backed my way up to where I went wrong and began over. I conceded that the other penalty points were correct, but not the extra 10-second penalty. Not to mention that I was the fastest of all the slalom racers, and that even with that 10-second penalty, I had lost by less than a second.

Well, she listened patiently to my explanation, took my copy of the slalom course and said she would take the information and get back to me. It took less than 5 minutes of sweating outside the tent before the officials came out and congratulated me on my victory. They had indeed given me an undeserved penalty. I was back to being on top of the world, but I wished I wouldn't keep making it difficult on myself.

At the medal presentation, the silver medalist from Korea congratulated me and said I deserved the gold. "You very fast", he smiled. Morice Hennessey from New Zealand was third. He wanted to swap team jackets, and I was more than happy to oblige. It's in my collection.

Competition on the track was stiff though, even if some of the big-name athletes were competing in Sweden. But the Canadian team was still plenty strong.

Paul Clark was dominate in his Class 2 events, while Chris Daw and Ron Robillard were winning medals in their classes. Only I seemed to be having difficulties. I removed both my steering handles and the compensator bar to render the device inoperable to enable my chair to pass inspection, but my difficulty in getting around the corners without losing speed continued. I knew my level of fitness was good enough to challenge for medals, but I realized it might not happen.

I wheeled an 18.4 in my semi-final of the 100, but it was not quick enough to make the final. I fared a little better in 400, wheeling a 1:15 in my heat, followed by a 1:12 in the semi-final. But my final run of 1:11 was only quick enough for fourth and not a personal best.

I finally had to admit that the chair was better suited to the road, and that I had some decisions to make moving forward. In the meantime, we still had the relays to wheel.

I was pencilled in for the 4 x 400 metres, along with Paul, Chris and Ron. Being the only one without a track medal, discounting my slalom gold, I was anxious for a better effort.

I led off and got a good jump at the gun, touching Paul with the team in third position. Away he went, as did Chris and Ron on their turn. The gap got shorter and shorter until the frontrunner was in Ron's rear-view mirror, and we wheeled to the gold in a time of 4:40.19. So, with a little help from my friends, I came home with another gold to go along with my slalom prize, ensuring my trip to Stoke was extra special.

But I was determined to have another track racer built from scratch. Paul was unstoppable in his 3-wheeled racer and there were enough other wheelers from around the world who were competing on 3-wheels, to convince me it was the chair of the future.

When I returned home, I had settled on two courses of action. I would corroborate with Doug once more, on what I hoped would be the ultimate track chair.

And while I could still use my road chair, its width would continue to rob me of power, even if I somehow stabilized my seating position. Short of literally cutting it in half, my only solution was another chair, perhaps the one I saw in Miami. And after some consideration, I took careful measurements, and I mean careful measurements, before I ordered the Top End chair I had seen in Florida.

The '87 Nationals in Brantford represented another big milestone in the advancement of wheelchair sports in Canada when the Canadian Forresters agreed to be the corporate sponsors for the next 3 national competitions. They would now be called the Canadian Forresters Games for the Disabled and would be held every other year going forward.

The Forresters were a fraternal Life Insurance company based in Brantford and they had committed to hosting the '87/'89/'91 Nationals. This was a big deal for us athletes in Canada since now we had ongoing sponsorship, instead of wondering each year if there would be funds for a national championship. It was another sign that disabled sports was coming of age.

These games were less than 2 weeks after coming back from England and I felt rather sluggish during the weekend. That resulted in a couple of silver and a couple of bronze medals when the dust had settled.

Chapter 17: Reaching for The Top

However, together with Paralympic veteran Ron Thompson, teammate Chris Daw and rookie Jeff Adams, we won both the 4 x 100 and the 4 x 400 metre relays to add to Ontario's gold medal total.

Something I was looking forward to though, was the slalom finals. Having won the provincials in front of a big crowd, and winning gold under pressure in England, I was hoping for the slalom trifecta, by adding the National title to my personal list.

The course was a one-run affair, and not near as complicated a course as the one in England, but it would be a good test, nonetheless. The gun sounded and off I went, but before I could reach the first pylon, my right front wheel hit a tiny pebble that had somehow found its way onto the course. Usually the course is swept clean, but there it was, and I pitched forward with my back wheels coming off the ground.

The natural reaction is to put your hand out to save yourself from going ass over teakettle, but that's dangerous during the slalom. With my hand outstretched toward the ground, I balanced on both my wheels for a split second before I bounced back on my rear wheels and continued around the pylon.

As I finished the first obstacle, I noticed out of the corner of my eye that a red flag had gone up. Damn I must have nicked the pylon going around it, but no problem. Keep going, and I did, touching nothing and making no more mistakes. Good as gold.

But before I could celebrate, I was called over by the head official and the official that threw the flag. I thought I had touched a pylon, costing me 3 seconds. But I had a big lead, so no worries. But the official had thrown the flag because she thought I had touched the ground with my hand before the chair righted itself, but she wasn't sure. The head official came over and asked me if I had touched the ground.

The head official was the great and dedicated Barb Montemurro, and we had known each other for over a decade, having gone to numerous provincial and international competitions together. Before she passed away, she would make her way into the Wheelchair Sports Hall of Fame for her decades of work, and on this day, she was going to give me the final say, disqualified or National Champion?

Ever since the question had been put to me, my mind had been replaying the sequence repeatedly. *Did I touch the ground?* I could see it in my mind's eye as my arm reached out in a natural reaction, to prevent a face-plant. I'm suspended on my front wheels for a moment... and as my fingernail brushes the surface, I'm back on four wheels heading for that first pylon.

I know that the brief contact did not prevent me from tipping over, and if I had fallen, I wondered if the pebble on the surface would have allowed me a restart. It all ran through my head. But regardless of whether I got a restart, I knew it could only go one way. My mind replayed the event over and over, and that sensation of my nail scraping the ground was always front and centre.

I knew that all the fun over the congratulations for winning would ultimately take a backseat to that little voice in my head that would be continually whispering "it was just a fingernail, just a fingernail". Rats... I hate that voice.

So, I copped to a guilty plea. "It was just the end of my fingernail, seriously, my fingernail, but technically I touched the ground", I lamented. So that was it, disqualified. No opportunity for a restart either. Plenty of congratulations for doing the right thing but gosh darn, no trifecta!

A couple of weeks later, Bev and I travelled to Owen Sound so that I could do a slalom competition as part of a fund-raising effort to aid Participation House. This was the same Organization that had benefited from the Wheels 'n' Heels road-race that I had entered in previous years. Bev and I were offered a night's stay at a local hotel, and I was an invited guest on the local radio station to talk about wheelchair sports. I said yes, and off we went.

Had a nice chat on the radio station the night before and I was looking forward to putting on a show. When we arrived at the site of the demonstration, however, we realized that the event was set up as a competition with a huge trophy sitting on the awards table.

One of the sponsors had gone undoubtedly overboard, because it reminded me of the karate awards you would see on TV, with the winner standing behind their 3-foot trophy.

As I contemplated the change, I noticed a couple of young boys, maybe 8 or 9, both with spina bifida I believe, who were checking out the awards when I showed up. I introduced myself and asked them if they were ready for the competition. They said they knew they had no chance against me, but they were determined to beat each other for the smaller trophy that was on the table. I said good luck and off I went.

The course was very easy with no hard obstacles. This was set up so that the kids could get through the course without too much trouble. Just a number of forward and backwards gates, and a small curb to jump up, and down the other side.

There was a small ceremony at the beginning and then the competition began. I tried to put on a good show, popping a wheelie and staying on just my back wheels as I made my way around the course, having fun.

When I was done it was time for the two boys to race. I enjoyed watching them working their way through the pylons, backing up slowly to get through the gates without touching anything.

Of course, it was no contest, and I was declared the winner. Up I went to the front to receive my trophy. I sat it on my lap and took the microphone to say thanks for putting on a great show. However, I said, since I am on the National team, I can't be accepting this award and that the trophy belongs to the young lad who came second.

What a laugh. The expression on both boys' faces was worth the price of admission. Now they both had hardware to take back home.

Everyone knew I made the story up, but they went along with the ruse. A little good goes a long way. Everyone went home happy, and I hoped perhaps one day in the future they would suit up for Canada. That would be something.

Back home again, all that was left in the year was to prepare for my two favourite marathons, Toronto, scheduled for the last Sunday in September and Detroit, a couple of weeks later. And I began to formulate what I wanted in the construction of my new track chair.

The day of the Toronto Marathon was cool but sunny as I found myself with Doug, Brien and the rest of the other wheelers on the start line for the marathon. For a change there was a half dozen racers lined up for the start, but my intention was to break at the gun and leave the rest of the field to fight it out with.

I took the lead from the start and didn't look back until I broke the tape in 2:20:55. Doug was second, but unknown to us, he hadn't bothered to register, so he was disqualified, and Brien took second prize instead.

Two weeks later, a bunch of us headed to Windsor for the Detroit Free Press Marathon. This would be the 3rd year in a row that I wheeled Detroit. I loved flying down that Windsor Tunnel. This particular year, once we had settled into our hotel rooms, we headed across the border into Detroit and fattened up in Greektown in preparation for the race the next day.

As usual, the marathon began with a race to the Windsor/Detroit Tunnel. Flying down the Tunnel is both exciting and challenging. To me, the tunnel was always the best part. I loved to go fast, and I never slowed myself down on a descent unless I had to make a corner at speed. Otherwise, I leaned forward and let it go.

I went out with the first group but by the time we reached the top of the Tunnel and onto the Detroit streets, I had fallen back. I kept a steady pace and tried to pick up my speed when I hit sections of smooth pavement, eventually joining a pack that I worked with to the finish line.

Philipe Couprie of France won the marathon with American Mike Trujillo second. I was 3rd in my Class, 10th overall, and finished in my fastest time at Detroit in 2:10:17.

My new Top End racing chair arrived from Florida soon after the Detroit Marathon and I wheeled out on the road as much as possible before the snow started falling. I took it on the track at Variety but using the compensator to get around the corners was the only way it would go around smoothly, so I was forced to use my HCM chair on the track until my new super-chair was ready.

When the 1987 edition of Run Barbados began to loom in December, I was pleasantly surprised when Ron Thompson called to say I had been offered another trip to Barbados for the 10K and marathon. The race director told him that the winners of the past two marathons were invited back. As well, a group of Americans, including the winner of the Invacare Cup, a US-based wheelchair road racing circuit, would be invited. The challenge of racing against a field of top-notch marathoners was going to be fun, and I was not going to turn down the opportunity to race in Barbados again and have an opportunity to lower my own personal time. And it would

Chapter 17: Reaching for The Top

be the first marathon in my new Top End racing chair, which meant I was about to wheel Barbados 3 years in a row in 3 different racing chairs.

The Canadian group consisted of Ron, Doug, Mark Johnson, Marnie Abbott and me. The US was represented by Mike Trujillo, Richard Hoyt and New Zealand's Robert Courtney, who had now made America his home. Also included was another great marathoner and multi-medal Games winner, the legendary Chris Hallam from Wales. This was going to be a fast race.

After we experienced another torrential downpour, just before the start of the 10K, the race was on. As expected, Courtney and Trujillo bolted right away, in hopes of creating a gap so that the two of them could draft off each other and leave the pack behind.

I had no chance of staying with that group, so I wheeled with the rest and tried to position myself to make it a sprint to the finish when the time came. That would be my best chance.

In the end Courtney had a quicker sprint and beat Trujillo to the tape. Ron was third, with Chris Hallam not far behind. I knew that once we turned the last corner, the finish line was not that far away, so I broke from the second pack just before the corner. Coming out of the turn, I got a jump big enough to prevented anyone behind me from catching me before the finish line.

I finished in 32:00. Fourth place and not my best time wheeling a 10K, but I was still getting used to the new chair. It did a much better job of absorbing the cobblestones and I had good speed rolling down the main road.

Having done the marathon twice, I had a good idea of what I would be facing before we lined up at Grantly Adams Airport. Since I had no intention of trying to stay with the front-runners, I had already decided to stay with the second group again and try and pull off the same strategy as I used for the 10K. Make it come down to a sprint. I figured it was my best bet.

I knew the Americans would use the same tactic against Ron and Chris in the marathon as they used in the 10k. They would jump ahead and take turns drafting each other to prevent anyone from joining.

By the results, I think they might have had other plans. The two of them left together, with Ron wheeling close behind and Chris Hallam a few yards back. The rest of us were content to take a slower pace and save something for the finish. No-one wanted to burn out. I had seen my share of rabbits.

Normally when you are drafting with one another, you need to be aware of your surroundings and the conditions of the road ahead. That's the responsibility of the pack leader, to alert those behind that he was about to move around something in the road. It's what you do if you're working together as a group. If you're not working together, well.

Luckily for the Americans, they saw the pothole and went around, whereas Ron did not and crashed. This time there would be no quick fix. They had pretty much taken him out. Chris Hallam had fallen off the pace just a bit and he was able to react to Ron's crash and go around.

By the time, our second group reached the same spot, Ron was preparing to be loaded into the van. We heard his version of the crash once we finished the race.

It wasn't long before I found myself pulling ahead, and because I felt the pace was too slow and the new chair was rolling smoothly, I decided to forge ahead alone. I had done this marathon twice on my lonesome and there were no surprises. If I didn't allow myself to overheat, I was fit enough to carry on alone. I wanted a faster time than the year before and I realized it would not be possible if I stayed at the pace we were going.

At the finish line, the previous day's results were reversed as Mike outsprinted Robert to the finish line, winning in 2:00:20. One second faster. Chris Hallam was third. That must have been a great finish to the marathon to witness. No-one had ever finished a marathon in Barbados in two hours. I worked hard until the end and crossed the line in 2:26:41.

Presentation ceremonies were great, as usual, and then we had another week of relaxing by the pool. Unfortunately, this time I was the one who had to go home early, and Bev got to hang with the guys. It was the last time I raced in Barbados but what a great experience.

Chapter 18:
Show's Over

Ever since I had come back from England, I had begun to formulate exactly how I wanted my new track chair to turn out. With my size and weight, and regardless of any wind that might slow me down, I still needed the lightest chair, with no unnecessary accessories to weigh me down if I was to be successful. And more importantly, I had to be as tight in the seat as possible.

I went into this partnership knowing that motivation would be the biggest challenge since my buddy Bill Brouse would not be there to lend his voice to keep the project on track. He had switched to playing basketball with the NWBA Kitchener Spinners full-time years ago, so I was on my own.

My former basketball teammate Dennis Kloppenburg had decided he was interested in a new chair as well. He had been racing for a few years, and he decided to help with our build. Though he wanted to see how mine turned out before he would commit himself.

But I felt the new design would be a big leap forward if it turned out the way I wanted. If I had hopes of producing podium worthy times once again, I needed a chair that fit me like a glove.

I knew that in the future all racing chairs would be 3-wheelers, and this new chair would only have one front wheel as well. The biggest difference was going to be in the design of the frame.

I wanted a molded fiberglass bucket seat, one that would hold me tightly in place and allow no lower body movement whatsoever. The bucket needed to be tight enough so that I could literally hang from a bar in the chair, with the wheels on, without sliding out.

The chair would be another T-frame design, comparable to that of the old 'SBS' chair we built in the early '80s, but I wanted to use a much smaller diameter tubing, and I wanted the bucket and the whole frame molded together and covered in fiberglass, so that it was one solid piece. I thought it would be plenty strong enough for my purpose. Then we'd finish off the front end with a custom 14" wheel/fork combination that would only track straight. I intended to use my hips to get around the corners.

Doug had already decided that this first chair would be one of many and he invested in a shop in Scarborough where he could do the work of building the chairs. It was his intention to start a business building racing chairs for a living. Mine would be number one.

My back-wheel setup for the new chair would be unique as well. After spending more than a few hours with Leo from LocalMotion and going through all the trick stuff that the racing bikes used, he had come up with a great idea.

Because of my weight, and since I only planned to race the chair on the track, he thought I could get away with using ultra-light 700cc velodrome rims. He also suggested using two different lengths of aero blade spokes. Instead of being rounded from one end to another, like regular spokes, aero spokes are flattened along the middle, enabling them to be more streamlined.

The shorter inside spokes, laced straight up and down, would get my wheels as close to the seat as possible. The longer spokes would be angled out and cross-laced. Wolber Profils tires would finish off the rear wheel combination.

I had not yet decided whether I was going to use the custom 'SBS' hubs or use a set of Phil Wood racing hubs that were now available on the market. I did decide to go with smaller diameter hand-rims to hopefully increase my top end speed, but I ordered these from Florida.

In late January, Dennis came over to the shop to help us pour the mold for the bucket. I assumed that all the instructions were read and followed as they mixed the chemicals together and in hindsight, I should have read them myself.

Chapter 18: Show's Over

We made a frame for me to sit in, using wood, cardboard and silver duct tape to make a rough shape of the mold and once I got settled in the proper position, they poured the mixture all around me.

As it began to react and expand, it also started to get hot, very hot indeed. I was only wearing my underwear and before long it started to get a mite uncomfortable. Then it began to get unbearable as my skin felt like it was on fire.

At one point I said, "Get me the **** out of here", but all I heard was "Five more minutes", so I grit my teeth and closed my eyes.

An hour into the ordeal, they finally cut me out. Chemical burns had turned my skin bright red, and my unmentionables…well…they were well done. The mold was fine though. Doug and Dennis were quite happy. It had better be worth it.

Once the snow melted, and even though I had my sights on Korea, I was still having fun wheeling in the various road races around Ontario. I met a lot of the same runners at these events, and they were always telling me about races that were flat and wheelchair friendly. I was looking forward to wearing my new race jersey in one of the upcoming events.

Over the years I have trained using many different methods to get fit, and to maintain that high level of fitness going forward. When Graham first began coaching me, interval training was the main component of my overall training regime in the early years when we were only racing up to the 1500 metre. Once I was spending a considerable amount of time out on the road, my training also consisted of Fartlek runs.

Fartlek runs are training sessions of a determined distance with a wide range of paces included. This helps during longer distances. The idea being that if someone made a break during the race, you were prepared to pick up your pace if needed or if you sensed weakness in your opponent, you would have the ability to up the tempo yourself.

Once I started spending considerable time on the roads and was wheeling marathons, I began to incorporate recovery runs as well. Recovery runs are intended to be slow and easy, usually following a long run or a hill/speed workout. Sometimes I would wheel a long run once a week at a moderate pace, followed by a rest day.

Just before Bev and I headed to Windsor for the Indoor Classic in February, Team Canada manager Barb Montemurro called to remind me of the importance of showing well in Windsor. I spent as much time as I could on the 200-metre track at Variety as I waited patiently for the chair to take shape, but I wasn't confident my HCM chair was up to the task.

I thought about using my new Top End chair on the track, but it was front-heavy and without the use of the compensator or steering handle, navigating the corners at speed would not be possible. I'd do the best I could with what I had. The future was promising, and I knew the new racer would turn heads when I unveiled it for the first time.

Windsor was just like I thought it was going to be, I was too slow in the corners. I was untouchable in the 60 metres but continued to lose ground on every lap. The results were not what I needed, but I was confident the new chair would be ready to roll before training camp.

At the end of February, I sat in the unfinished bucket for the very first time. It was tight, that's for sure. The thickness of one pair of track pants took up all the space once I sat in it. The seat stuck to me like Lycra. Step one complete. There was still a lot to do.

When I closed my eyes, I could see myself in the finished project flying around the track, but it was hard waiting for it to be finished. After 2 months, we had managed to build the bucket. At this rate I was beginning to worry the chair would not be finished in time and my last chance to wear Canada's colours would evaporate.

While I waited for the chair to be completed, the new set of rear wheels I ordered from Leo at LocalMotion were ready for pickup. Since the new chair was far from finished, I planned to use them on my HCM frame in hopes they would somehow help me shave a second off my elapsed times.

Leo also hooked me up with a heart rate monitor that included a stopwatch with clock and lap functions. It was the first chair I had with electronics on board.

Near the end of March, I wheeled the Around the Bay 30K in Hamilton. This race is the oldest road race in North America, having its inaugural run in 1894. The trophy for winning is unbelievable huge, old and beautiful. Having your name on that would be quite the honour.

Chapter 18: Show's Over

The Ontario Road race co-ordinator at the time, Al Brooks, told me about this race, but said it had a very steep corkscrew incline up an access road that he was not sure someone in a wheelchair would be able to climb. But I entered anyway. I love a challenge and the chance to be the first wheeler in such a historic race was too much to turn down.

On race-day, the temperature was just above freezing, but with the wind gusting from 37 to 50 Km per hour, the wind chill was minus 13 C. This was going to be a test of attrition. Just to finish would be a good enough challenge.

The incline was tough indeed, steep enough that it forced me to push off my tires instead of my hand-rims. And steep enough that even with my chest pressed against my knees I was very close to flipping over backwards. That position forced me to climb, or should I say crawl, up to the main road. It wasn't all that long, maybe 50 metres max, but energy sapping for sure. My arms were trembling by the time I reached the top.

Took me awhile to shake off the effects of the climb, but the rest of the way was relatively smooth. The chair worked fine on the road, and I would end up being the first wheelchair athlete to complete this historical race.

There were 1,216 at the starting line but only 1,120 made it to the end. I finished in 1:50:26, good for 20th place, and I was looking forward to tackling the course another time.

At the end of the month, I wheeled a 200 and 400 metre time trial for coach Anthony Clegg at Variety Village, and he was concerned that there had not been much improvement in my times from Windsor. That's because I had been spending too much time trying to ensure the build of my racer kept moving forward. My partner had a great mind, but he did more *thinking* than *doing*.

I hoped this super chair project was not going to be my undoing. Korea would surely be my last chance to race on the track for Canada. I didn't feel a lot of anxiety at the time, since I hoped my gold medal in the slalom from last year's World Championships would help cash my ticket overseas, but you never know. The slalom was a major event in Asia, and I sure wanted the chance to defend my title.

In early April, Bob Ellery and I were contacted at War Amps by a representative from the Canadian Wheelchair Sports Association. They were hoping we would attend a demonstration of wheelchair racquetball, that they were going to put on at the Toronto Airport Racquetball Club. Sounded like fun, and they thought that my being involved in the slalom might make me a good candidate to try out racquetball. Maybe this would prolong my involvement in wheelchair sports, so we took them up on the invitation.

What a blast I had. This was a sport I liked. The rules were virtually the same as able-bodied racquetball, except, like wheelchair tennis, the rules gave us two bounces instead of one. If ever there was a wheelchair sport that merged seamlessly with its able-bodied counterpart, tennis was it, and racquetball seemed to be a close second. The only barrier was the small door to get onto the court, but once the back wheels were popped off the chair and put back on once you were inside, you were good to go.

The president of the National Wheelchair Racquetball Association at the time was BC's Dave Hinton. Although able-bodied, he sat in a wheelchair for the demonstration, and hardly moved, though he had me streaking all over the court trying to hit that little blue ball. It was the first lesson I learned: being fast certainly helped, but proper positioning could make it look almost easy.

With the degree of strength Bob had in his hands, due to his level of disability, holding the racquet proved to be too difficult to be effective, so he was not interested moving forward. But over the summer I continued to travel to the Airport Club and was fortunate enough to be introduced to Eddie Khan. Knowing nothing about the history of racquetball I was surprised in the beginning that whenever anyone asked me who my coach was, as soon as I said Eddie Khan, their eyes would light up. I quickly found out that the Khan clan were famous in the sport of racquetball.

Didn't take me long to understand why. During our first training sessions together, like Ken Hinton had done to me before, Eddie had me racing all over the court. Not only that, but Eddie took it up a notch and instead of a wheelchair, he sat on a kitchen chair in the middle of the court, still able to reach all my shots and send me chasing around like a dog after a bone.

Chapter 18: Show's Over

I convinced a half dozen of my buddies to come out and try the sport, and by the end of the year there were eight of us that played at the Airport club.

We got our first taste of competition when the Club hosted the Provincial Singles Racquetball Tournament. Dennis beat me 3-2, to claim the first Provincial Championship.

May 1st saw me out on the road, once again trying to win the Hamilton Marathon and lay claim to the Provincial Championship. Despite my best effort, I remained the bridesmaid once more as Ron Robillard broke the tape first.

My new Top End chair felt solid on the road. Although it was heavier than my HCM chair, it fit me much better and there was no body movement during the race. It took corners at speed with no problem and steering was comfortable. The compensator kept me on a straight line whenever I needed it. I thought it was a good chair to help me lower my personal bests.

I received a letter from CWSA soon after, informing me that our Paralympic trials would coincide with the Nabob Nationals that would be held in Edmonton June 8th until the 12th.

In the meantime, I had to decide if I want to enter the Open 1500 metre time trial. At stake was a berth in the field of racers that were going to Belgium. The fastest wheelers in the world were going there for a chance to be one of the 8 athletes chosen to race in another exhibition 1500, this time at the Seoul Olympics. I had no illusions of being competitive against a field of our best, let alone the rest of the world, and so I politely declined.

I was also told the slalom was not going to be an event in Edmonton, so I assumed that I would be pencilled in for that event in Korea without having to qualify.

As I prepared to race in the Toronto Provincials, my new chair was still far from finished. While the bucket had been molded to the T-frame, it was still not even sanded smooth, and the front end had yet to be built. I was beginning to worry. So little time and so much still to do.

My fitness level was high though, and despite wheeling in the old frame, my new wheels worked great, and I managed to race to victory in my four events and added the slalom crown to finish off a good weekend.

But there was still concern all around. Being unbeatable in Ontario was one thing. If my times were not vastly different in Edmonton I would be in serious trouble. I was not going to be fast enough, regardless of my training, to put down times that would be competitive internationally without the new chair under me. I was beginning to cross my fingers, a lot.

Ontario team coach Anthony Clegg called just before we left for Edmonton for the Nationals in June to say the slalom was not going to be an event offered in Korea. I found that hard to believe since it was a big deal in that part of the world, but it was bad news regardless.

But not near as bad as boarding a plane for Edmonton a couple of weeks later with my new chair still unfinished. I had been training hard, but I was still a good 2 seconds per lap slower than what I should be. I didn't want to hear excuses as to why it wasn't finished. The damage had already been done.

To make matters worse, when we arrived in Edmonton, we were classified yet again. A new world classification system would be introduced after Korea, but it still had implications leading up to the competition. Depending upon your new classification and the odds of medalling going forward, a choice had to be made before then.

Do you take a veteran with an outside chance of a track medal but not being in the team's next 4-year plan, or do you take someone else for the experience they will get and worry about medals later?

This time classification pegged me as a T53 in the new system, and with the competition I knew I would now be facing, the hill suddenly became much harder to climb.

Through the week I battled as hard as I could. In my heart I assumed this would be the last time I'd be at the Canadian Nationals, and I wanted to leave nothing on the table. Not having the new chair to compete in and then being reclassified, put me in a rather foul mood to say the least, but I emptied the tank and finished with 4 silvers to add to my personal total. I went faster than I had all year, but would Korea be in my future?

Once back in Ontario, I did everything, and I mean everything, to advance the build, but the call that I had been dreading for months finally came. Anthony called in early July to inform me that I did not make the team for Korea. Just not fast enough in my old chair. And although I did get a call a week later from Barb and team coach Mari Ellery telling me to

Chapter 18: Show's Over

keep training hard just in case an opening appeared, I knew I was done. Not happy was putting it mildly.

With news that I was not going to Korea, the building process ground to a stop. What was the hurry? Now we had the rest of the year to "fine tune" the chair into something spectacular. Whatever. The only thing left for me to do was head out on the road for the rest of the year. I had some steam to blow off, and the road was a great place to do it.

The weather for the September Toronto Marathon was excellent, not much wind and the temperature comfortable for wheeling. I felt strong, it was time for a personal best. We had more than a half dozen entrants for a change and everyone was primed to have a good time.

I was not in a good mood to start the race though. A couple of days earlier I had been at the Airport Racquetball club practising with Coach Khan when Dennis came by for practise. He was surprised to find out that I was unaware that the frame of the new chair had cracked a month ago. Bad enough it wasn't ready for Korea, but to break the frame and not tell me?

When the gun went off, I put the hammer down immediately and attempted to leave the field behind. The Toronto Marathon had changed the racecourse on more than one occasion, so it was difficult to beat your own personal time when the terrain changed year to year, but I wanted to be out there with my own thoughts as I wheeled down the road.

I had a good 200 yards of real estate between me and the rest of the pack, and I was just beginning to turn right onto another street when I saw something out of the corner of my eye.

I had time to close my eyes before the bike rider hit me broadside and we both crashed into the curb. He flew off his bike and knocked me out of my chair on our way to the pavement. He had ignored the policeman who was directing traffic and thought he could get across the intersection before the pack he saw up the road, would reach him. He never saw me until the last moment.

We were both scrapped up, him more than me, since he flew a lot farther. My biggest concern was the state of my chair. My right back wheel had a broken spoke, but the left wheel had lost more than a couple and the hand-rim was bent out of shape. With help, I got back into the chair.

Once I was ready to roll again, I left the guy sitting on the curb to ponder the destruction my chair had done to his bike, as I tried to catch up to the field. I had a long stretch of road facing me and no-one was in sight. I had been still gathering my wits about me when the pack of wheelers had gone past, so I had no idea how far back I was. Time to play catch-up.

I kept rolling. The wheels were protesting on every revolution they made and as the miles wore on, I would hear a "ping" and another spoke would let go. Time was running out.

In the beginning, people offered me encouragement as I passed by. Since everyone else had gone by minutes earlier, I suspect they were more "pity cheering" for the poor bugger limping along, and not realizing his chair was self destructing as he wheeled. But I appreciated the gestures, nonetheless.

However, a marathon is a long race and I kept pushing, trying not to put too much pressure on my damaged hand-rim. I had completed every marathon I had entered at that point, and I was determined to reach the finish line if nothing else.

Eventually I caught the pack of wheelers, and that left just one competitor, off in the distance. Doug had decided to leave the pack and head out on his own, so I picked up my pace. I didn't want the wheel to completely collapse before the finish line after all the work it took to get that far, but last thing I wanted to do was to come in second, considering the circumstances.

I was closing the distance, but unfortunately, he was tipped off. A bike rider who had passed me, must have told him that someone was gaining on him, because he picked up his pace.

It was more than I could duplicate without taking the real chance of breaking more spokes and having the wheel completely fold up. I let him go and settled for second place.

My favourite number has been 21 for a long time, years before I began racing and it has produced both lucky and seriously unlucky results in the past. So, I had to smile when I saw that my finishing time was 2:21:21. Doug was quite happy with his time of 2:19:0, since it was a personal best, and the first and last time he beat me in a race.

Chapter 18: Show's Over

A couple of weeks later, a group of us headed down to Windsor to once again tackle the Detroit Free Press Marathon. I had a good wheel. I went out with the initial pack and even passed the eventual winner going down the tunnel. But staying with the main pack for that initial push to the tunnel took a lot out of me, as did climbing the incline onto US soil.

So, once we emerged from the Tunnel, I was left behind, but I wheeled with another pack and finished in 2:22:54, ending up 11th out of the 45 wheelers who entered.

It was good enough. I was wheeling on old wheels and hand-rims, since the bike shop was not able to get me a new set of wheels put together in time to replace the destroyed pair.

The race was won by Doug Wight in a new course record of 1:50:02. Fellow American Dutch Martin broke the tape in second. I never imagined anyone being able to finish a marathon in under 2 hrs, and yet years later, marathoners would wheel under 1:15:00!

While I never made the Seoul Paralympics, I was eager to find out the results and see how Canada had done. More than a couple of notable Canadian athletes were absent, but we still had a good group of veterans, athletes that were aiming to continue their success, and rookies just getting their feet wet.

From the super quick 100 metre to the energy-sapping marathons and beyond, wheelers continued to push the limit as the chairs got more sophisticated. As did training methods and everything else that could produce results.

Korea was significant in that the three-wheeled chair was now legal going forward, but mechanical steering was still banned.

The Korean Paralympics were the first Games in 24 years that were held in the same host country as the Olympics. With a team of 79 athletes, Canada was second to the American contingent of 195. Australia brought 76 competitors.

Looking back on the '84 results for a comparison proved to be quite interesting. Three of our six big guns, Class 4's Rick Hansen and Ron Minor and Class 5 Mel Fitzgerald had retired after tremendous careers on the National team. While Andre Viger, Paul Clark and Dan Westley were still on the team, it was our quad team that had vastly improved in the 4 years since the last Games.

In '84, Terry Gehlert, a 1B racer from Saskatchewan won the bronze in the 100 final in England, and that was the lone medal that the group brought home. In Korea, they captured at least one medal in almost every race offered at these Games.

In Class 1A, it was mostly a battle among German countrymen Hans Lubbering, Gunther Obert and Heinrich Koeberle. Between the three of them, they won all the Class 1A races.

Class 1B was dominated by a pair of Canadians, Serge Raymond and Clayton Gerein. Between them, they won every event except the 100 which was won by Peter Carruthers of Great Britain. Serge won the 200, Clayton won the 400 and 800. Serge won the 1500, Clayton won the 5,000, and Serge finished off winning the 1B marathon.

While Canadian Andre Beaudoin won a gold in the 200, silver in the 100 and 400, and a bronze in the 800, the top dog of Class 1C was American Jeff Worthington who was victorious in the 400 – 800 – 1500 and 5,000 metre races, while teammate John Brewer won the 1C marathon.

The Class 2 battle was a more wide-open affair as 5 different athletes collected multiple medals. Germany's Errol Marklein ruled the sprints, winning gold in the 100 - 200 and 400 and a bronze in the 5,000. Canada's Paul Clark won gold in the 800 and a silver in the 1500. The great Swiss racer, Hans Frei won the 1500 and the 10,000. Germany's Wolfgang Peterson took the gold in the 5,000. Canada's Marc Quessy won a silver in the 100 and then ran away from the field in winning the Class 2 marathon. Teammate Paul Clark won the marathon silver.

Lars Lofstrom of Sweden and Belgium's Paul van Winkle would both win 5 medals each in Class 3 competition. Lofstrom won gold in the 200 and the 1500, silver in the 100 and the 800 and a bronze in the 400. Van Winkle was victorious in the 400, the 800, and 5,000, with a silver in the 200 and 1500.

Germany's Robert Figl won the 100, took silver in the 400 and a bronze in the 200. Gregor Golombeck of Germany won the 10,000, won a silver in the 5,000 and a bronze in the 1500 final.

Chapter 18: Show's Over

Canada's Andre Viger got into the action once the distances lengthened, winning a bronze in the 800 and 1500, silver in the 5,000 and gold in the marathon.

In Class 4, Hee Sang Yu of Korea won the 100 and Jan Kleinheerenbrink of the Netherland took home the 200 before a pair of Frenchmen took over.

First up, Farid Amarouche won the 400, the 1500 and 5,000, with silvers in the 800 and 10,000. Countryman J P Poitevin took gold in the 10,000 and a silver in the 1500 and 5,000. They would work together in the marathon with Amarouche winning the gold and Poitevin the silver. American Rafael Ibarra won the bronze.

Korean Bong Ho Lee won the 100 and then Class 5/6 was ruled by Switzerland's Franz Nietlispach, who cleared the table, winning 5 gold in the 200 - 400 – 800 – 1500 and 5,000.

Once Nietlispach was parked, it was time for others to play. Bronze medalist in the 5,000, van Breemen of the Netherlands won the 10,000 gold. Jon Puffenberger of the US won the silver and Nezar Ahmed of Kuwait took home the bronze. The Class 5/6 marathon was won by American Jon Puffenberger, with countryman Tom Foran winning the silver to go with the same medal he won in '84. George Schrattenecker of Australia won the bronze.

Canadian double amp Dan Westley was not wheeling in his usual wheelchair division in these Paralympics but was entered in the amputee division of the wheelchair races.

Almost the entire set of events for the amp racers came down to the efforts of three individuals, Canada's Dan Westley, France's Mustapha Badid and Sweden's Hakan Ericsson. The three battled at every distance.

Dan won the 100, the 800 and took silvers in the 200, 400, 1500 and 5,000. Mustapha took home gold in the 200, 1500 and 5,000 and a silver in the 100. Hakan won gold in the 400, a silver in the 800 and bronze in the 100 and 200.

Badid ruled the road as well, bring home the gold in the marathon, with Canada's Ted Vince winning the marathon bronze.

After the 88 Paralympics in Koreas were over, a group of our marathoners went to the 8th Oita Marathon in Japan. The race was won by Paul Clark in 1:38:27 with countryman Andre Viger less than a second behind in 1:38:31. Bo Lindkvist of Sweden was third with Canadians Marc Quessy and Luke Gingras fourth and fifth.

Once again, wheelchair athletes put on track demonstrations at the 88 Olympics in Korea. Unlike the 1984 exhibition 1500 metre race where Paul van Winkle raced out to the front and stayed there, the '88 contest was a tight thrilling race that came down to the wire.

This time Mustapha Badid of France nipped Paul by one tenth of a second, stopping the clock at 3:33.51. American Craig Blanchette was in third in 3:34.37.

Farid Amarouche of France, Gregor Golombek of Germany, Andre Viger of Canada, Robert Figl of Germany and Hee Sang Yu of Korea rounded out the field.

The women's 800 exhibition race was won by American Sharon Hendricks in 2:11.49, defeating Connie Hansen of Denmark and fellow American Candace Cable-Brooks.

Chapter 19: Change of Pace

Over the winter and into the new year, I entered a few racquetball tournaments in preparation for the National Racquetball Championships that were going to be held at the Toronto Airport Club in February. With wheelchair racquetball fully integrated with its able-bodied counterpart, the best wheelchair racquetball players, would be converging on Toronto. I was looking forward to playing new opponents instead of the same guys all the time.

Since Dennis won the provincials the year before, he was entered in the "A" division and the rest of us local players were in the "B" division during the championships. Most of our competition came from a group of players from Manitoba who made the trip East.

It was a fun tournament and we had lots of spectators watching our matches. I got on a roll early and kept squeaking out victories as the tournament progressed.

Once the weekend competitions were over, and I had survived an accidental smash to my ear during the final, I had defeated Manitoba's John Breen for the National "B" Division crown. I followed Coach Khan's advice to the letter, but it was still unexpected and therefore even more fun. I was thinking this might be a sport I could be successful in moving forward.

Once March arrived it was time for the Around the Bay 30K road race once more. I took strange pleasure in climbing that brutal corkscrew incline that was part of the course. At the start line it was minus 15C with wind gusts of 30-40 km hour.

At the gun, marathoner Mark Johnson and I took off down the road. The wind made it hard to wheel and it became more a test of endurance than a road race. In the end I broke the tape in 1:48:18, good for 19th overall. Not my best time, but a couple of minutes faster than last year.

Later in the month I entered the Burlington/Coca-Cola 25K. The new Top End chair continued to work well, and I crossed the line in 1:26:25. Since there was no wheelchair division, I won the male 35-39 category, which did not sit well with the able-bodied runner who would have won had I not entered. The organizers promised there would be a wheelchair class in the next year's race, and there was.

A week later, I lined up at the start line for the Hamilton International Marathon. I wheeled a strong race, the chair worked great, and I finally rolled across the finish line ahead of the pack. I was a bridesmaid no more.

When the Nepean Ontario Games rolled around, I entered out of habit, I guess. Figuring my days on the national track team were over, I just wanted to be able to say I competed in all 15 Ontario Games for the Disabled, and the 3 previously named Provincial Wheelchair Games before I retired for good.

Held in the middle of June, I did all right in my five races, but didn't realize that I was now officially in the Master Class for all events moving forward, and so received another five gold medals for my races over the weekend.

I had come to the realization that they were now nothing more than participation medals, since they were not my idea of a gold medal. Don't get me wrong, I was glad my results enabled me to make the team going to the nationals once again, but based on my recent results, I harboured no dreams of coming back with a track medal. With the racing chair project called off for good, I'd have to wheel in my old HCM chair.

The fact that the slalom was back as an event at the nationals after a one-year banishment, made the prospect of going west important at least. If nothing else, I was determined to keep my national slalom crown when I retired.

I made the Ontario team going to Richmond BC for the '89 National Forresters Games for the Disabled, and true to my word, I wheeled a penalty free race and retired as National slalom champion for the ninth time. I even

Chapter 19: Change of Pace

managed a surprise bronze in the 100, by anticipating the gun and getting a good jump on the field, before my lead evaporated.

No such luck in my other races, but Ontario had a strong relay team, and we won the 4 x 100 metre relay. It was my last gold medal at the Canadian Nationals.

After competing in a local road race later in the summer, one of the runners asked me if I would ever consider wheeling a longer distance than the marathon. A race called the Dofasco/Golden Horseshoe 50-Miler was scheduled for October.

It was a road course that wound its way through the surrounding countryside around Hamilton, and it was 50 miles long. Fifty miles? That *would* be a challenge. One I was up for. Finishing the race was my priority, of course, since to anyone's knowledge no Canadian wheelchair athlete had competed in a 50-mile road race, and I had no intention of stopping until I rolled over the finish line.

With a chance to be the first wheelchair athlete to enter the event, I contacted Ed Alexander, the race director and asked him if I could enter. With the go-ahead behind me I began to prepare for the challenge.

The race began at the Tim Horton's Donut shop at the intersection of Highway 20 and Mud Street. As usual, there were numerous water stations along the route for the runners, but I couldn't stop of course for fear of getting my gloves wet and losing grip. To compensate during marathons, I had a water bottle mounted down by my feet. A flexible tube was taped to my leg and long enough that I could sip fluids as I wheeled along. Bev rode her bike along with me as well, carrying extra tires and a pump in case I had a flat along the way.

Early in the race, we were faced with an enormous hill that everyone was forced to climb. The hill was so long and so steep that many of the runners walked up the hill backwards to prevent themselves from injuring an Achilles tendon during the climb. Steep enough that I had to push off my tires and so long that I eventually developed a large blister on my back where it had rubbed on the back of my seat. It bled for the rest of the race and my back was a bit of a mess once I eventually rolled over the finish line.

But I carried on and the miles melted away until I reached another obstacle. The paved road turned into one covered in loose gravel, which is probably the worst surface you could possibly have for wheeling on. At one point a car came by to check on the athletes' well-being during the race. It was near the end, and I was wheeling on fumes, and I told them none too politely what I thought of a three-mile slog through this type of terrain.

Regardless, I pushed on and thankfully the road eventually became smooth, and I made a push for the finish line. I rolled through the tape in 6:58:22, good for second overall. Able-bodied ultra-marathoner Frank Vreezen of Burlington won in 6:41:0. It was a great experience, and I was assured that next year's race would be nothing but paved roads.

One of the cool things about this race was that it did not present a trophy to the winner. Instead, you received a great sweatshirt with the Dofasco / Golden Horseshoe 50-Miler logo on the front, and the #1 above the heart. I was presented with the #2 sweatshirt, but I had already decided that I would love to win this race and have that neat #1 for my memorabilia collection.

After the ceremonies were finished, I was informed that when the results were posted, I would be recognized as the first Canadian wheelchair athlete to complete a 50-mile road race. That was nice of them. More reason to return for another chance at that cool sweatshirt.

As usual, I wheeled the Toronto and Detroit Free Press Marathons. It was cold and windy for the Toronto race, but I wasn't really challenged, stopping the clock at 2:20:55.

The weather in Detroit a week later wasn't much better and I ended up with almost the same time, rolling over the finish line in 2:20.43. I finished on top in the Class 3 group and received a nice plaque as Top Canadian for finishing ahead of the other 8 countrymen who had entered the marathon.

In the late Fall of '89, marathon racer Andre Viger addressed the National Symposium for Coaches of Physically Disabled Athletes held in Richmond B.C. to explain and promote the new state-of-the-art racing wheelchair he had helped develop in conjunction with a company called Sodev from Rock Forest, Quebec. Along with fellow Quebec athletes Marc

Chapter 19: Change of Pace

Quessy and Serge Raymond, they had just begun using this unique state-of-the-art racing wheelchair called the V2.

Sodev was a research and development firm that also manufactured scientific instruments and other mechanical and electrical devises. The designer, Patrick Picker was an award-winning inventor and between his building skills and Andre's experience in racing, they came up with an amazing 3-wheeled racing chair, that was revolutionary in design and outfitted with many special features.

The most amazing thing to me was that it was not welded together like every other racing chair in the world but consisted of aircraft aluminum tubes that were joined together with high-strength plastic couplings. Armed with a screwdriver or an Allen key, it was possible to adjust your bucket to fit perfectly without effecting the wheel alignment in any way. From a practical point of view, it meant if you crashed and broke a regular welded chair during training or competition, there would be a lot of scrambling to get it repaired in time. With this system, the damaged parts could be swapped out for new ones.

Another great feature was the chair's ability to change the inclination of its rear wheels by a good margin, and yet not change the distance between the top of the wheels. In most other chairs, the camber of the back wheels is permanently welded at a degree chosen by the athlete.

Built almost entirely of aluminum alloys, it was super light and looked cool, but that was just the tip of the iceberg in terms of advanced technology. With no forks on the front wheel, the system employed a steering axis within the hub and instead of the usual piston system, the V2 used a cam devise that reduced friction and returned the wheel to its original position.

Another unique feature was its steering compensator that allowed you to adjust the tracking of your front wheel on sloped roads, or for going around the corners of a track. By dialing in the corners, you could go down the back stretch, tap the steering knob with your hand and the front wheel would turn and lock into that precise turning radius. Hitting the button on the other side coming out of the corner would straighten out the wheel to its original position. On the track it was a smooth transition into the corners and back out again. And it helped tremendously on the road where you might encounter miles of sloped roadway that would put a lot of strain on one arm to push straight.

My good friend and training buddy, Gino Vendetti found out about the V2 before I did, and he was in the process of ordering one and becoming the Ontario rep when he told me about the chair. Once I got a glimpse of the machine, I knew it was revolutionary to say the least, and I wanted one for myself.

Since Korea, the racing chair had begun to evolve once more. Nearly all the top racers were competing in a 3-wheeled chair of some type. If I harbored any thoughts of still racing on the track, I would have to have the best equipment and be the best shape of my life.

We drove to Quebec in November to get fitted and stayed the night as the guests of Mr. Picker and his wife. It was fascinating to see how the chair was built. If only I was twenty years younger.

Chapter 20: Three-Wheelers

In January of 1990, the sport of wheelchair road racing reached new heights in Australia, when the Quantas Oz Day 10K included an international field of world class road racers for the first time. The idea and success of this event was due to the efforts of Aussie world class marathoner Peter Trotter. He wheeled marathons all over the world and had represented Australia at numerous international competitions.

Fifteen wheelers comprised the Men's Open category, with 7 ladies in the Women's Open. Four junior athletes, four Master athletes over 40 and 7 racers in the Quad division, rounded out the field.

Seven nationalities were represented in the Men's Open, with athletes from Canada, Australia, Sweden, Belgium, Wales, Switzerland and the USA.

In a photo finish, American Craig Blanchette nipped Sweden's Bo Lindkvist at the wire, winning the 10K by 3/100th of a second in 23:55. Paul van Winkel of Belgium was third and Canada's Andre Viger was 4th.

The women's race was won by Ingrid Lauridsen of Denmark in 28.43.5 and the legendary Jan-Owe Mattsson easily won the Quad division in 31:00.3.

In March, I entered the Hamilton's Around the Bay 30K road race. This time I wheeled alone.

Like the year before it was cold. The temperature hovered around O C and with winds gusting up to 60 Km per hour, it wasn't surprising that of the 1,016 runners that started, over 130 would not finish.

The Top End racer was a very stable chair, but it had a much different feel to it though. Hard to describe, but it reminded me of the difference between the way a front-wheel car goes around corners, as opposed to a car with rear-wheel drive. However, it was my fastest time ever for the course, finishing in 1:46:45, good for 16th overall.

In the middle of April, my new Sodev racer arrived from Quebec. Remarkable was a good description of the V2. It was the most high-tech racer I would ever own, and I still have a blast flying down hills in the chair, even after all the years that have passed.

Statistically the chair came with one 16" Sun Metal Industries racing front wheel / steering axis within the hub / adjustable curve tracking mechanism / spring-cam device on steering bar /and adjustable rear wheel camber. The chair set me back $2,700, since I didn't have sponsors anymore, but the money was well spent. It fit like a glove and rolled as smooth as can be.

By now, Gino and I were members of the newly named Phoenix Track Club. After Ben Johnson had tested positive at the '88 Olympics, the club that he belonged to, tried to distance itself from the incident and from the "ashes", the Phoenix track club was born. This meant that we were part of the first able-bodied track and field club that included wheelchair athletes.

As well as the two of us, the club included wheelchair athletes Laura Misciagna, Keith Brettell and Martin Larocque. We were coached by the tandem of Kelly McCloud and Randy Marsh, and our first official competition as members of the Club was the Florida Sunshine Games in Tampa. Gino and I were looking forward to rolling the V2 out onto the track.

April weather in Florida was excellent and wheeling along effortlessly in the new chair brought a smile to my face. It garnered a lot of attention on the track since it was a new and completely unique machine. The chair was so smooth and once I dialed in the track's corners with the V2's tracking device, the chair went around the corners like it did when I used to steer my chair using my hand back in the '70's.

The first race in the new chair was an Open 800 metre. The race featured a good field of competitors, none better than legendary American, George Murray.

I finished second, but happy with my result. There had not been a lot of time to get in shape before the snow was gone, and most of the athletes at this competition, like George, lived in Florida or at least somewhere warm, so they didn't have to stop wheeling through the winter months. But it was a good shake-down run.

Later in the day, I wheeled an Open 400 and rolled in third. Again, I was satisfied with the result considering the competition and the amount of time I had wheeling in the new chair.

At the end of the month and back home again, I took the V2 out on the road for the first time to wheel the Burlington / Coca-Cola Classic 25k Road Race once again. Last year I wheeled it alone but this time I was joined by local marathoner Mark Johnson in the newly created wheelchair division. I broke the tape in 1:23:06.

The chair rolled effortlessly on the road. Going downhill in my tuck position, the steering handle was positioned so that I was able to use either hand or both, depending upon the situation, to steer around any obstacles I would encounter. I was liking it more and more.

In July, I entered the Ontario Games for the Disabled for the 16th and last time. With the V2 under me, I thought I might be able to give the young guns a run for their money. I fared all right, but since most of my time was now spent wheeling on the road, I hadn't done much track work and it showed.

Once I dialed the corners in, using the V2 patented steering system, I went around the bends with no problem. Good enough to win gold in the Master category, but not fast enough for a national team spot consideration.

However, I was still enjoying playing racquetball and I was looking forward to making the provincial team. Over the years, wheelchair racquetball had expanded quickly, much like tennis did years earlier and many people in the sport felt it had progressed to the point that it should be recognized as a medal event at the Stoke Games, as well as having a recognized Division in the able-bodied sport of racquetball.

At the Stoke Mandeville Games back in '87, Canadian Charles Drouin of the Canadian Wheelchair Sports Association continued the lobbying that he had began the previous year, to make wheelchair racquetball truly recognized.

Charles was at the Pan Am Games in Halifax in '82 and in England in '84 as the team's archery coach, and at the time was the Technical Coordinator for the Quebec Archery Federation. But he was relentless in his pursuit of seeing wheelchair racquetball officially recognized as a legitimate sport with all the advantages that distinction brought to the sport.

On Aug 2, 1990, wheelchair racquetball finally came of age on the international stage when the sport received not one but two international endorsements, with rights on inclusion in major games competitions. Both the Stoke Mandeville Wheelchair Sports Federation (ISMWSF) and the International Racquetball Federation (IRF) independently granted these rights. Congratulations to Charles Drouin for a job well done.

Unfortunately, playing racquetball became a lot more difficult due to events that were ultimately, out of my control. The main reason was that many of the guys that played the game travelled to Toronto from out of town and most decided it was not worth the effort. That only left 4 or 5 of us and due to an unfortunate incident that arose at the club, the number was significantly reduced once more.

The Airport Club backed up against the Park 'n Fly parking lot, and if you wanted to have a few beers or something, all the Club's members parked in the back and partied before heading inside. As a nice gesture for the wheelchair players, the Club designated a couple of wheelchair parking spots out front, so we didn't have to slog through the snow during the winter and spend time drying our chairs off before we could wheel onto the wood floors of the racquetball courts.

One day a few of the guys parked in wheelchair parking and began to party, instead of going out back first. When management realized what was going on, the guys were confronted regarding their behaviour. Without apologies forthcoming, they were all kicked out of the club and that left only John Klis and I. Trying to co-ordinate times when we were both free, became an issue and we didn't get to the Club very often. Once Bev and I moved out to Oshawa, the logistics became too difficult, and I stopped playing altogether.

In September I fulfilled the promise to myself that I would tackle the Dofasco/Golden Horseshoe 50-Miler once again and I talked Gino into doing the race as well. With both of us riding in our new V2 racers, we were all set to go.

Chapter 20: Three-Wheelers

Unfortunately, just as the race was about to begin, I realized I had locked all the gear Bev was going to carry during the race, in the van. I had no choice but to take off without her when the gun sounded and hope she would catch up. Within the first half hour of wheeling, she rode up beside me and we cruised along together, with Gino not far behind.

As promised, it was a different course than the year before, and there were no surprises. No brutal hill to climb and no stretches of loose gravel. Wheeling in the V2 was great. The miles past without incident. I finished in 6:50:28 and I got to put on that coveted # 1 sweatshirt.

The 1990 edition of the London Marathon in England that year was memorable, not for a record-breaking pace but for winning by controversial means. Everyone had been drafting one another on the road for years by now. Ever since we realized the benefits of having the wind blocked for you by the racer in front, it had been an acceptable practise, but with some unwritten rules. Teammates often took turns drafting off each other, to create a gap away from the field or to prevent another competitor from just tagging along. That was an acceptable practise.

Many times, a pack of five or six wheelers would take turns breaking the wind. However, if an athlete didn't take his turn, he might not get the heads-up about a pothole in the road and find himself eliminated from the equation.

Now I have been in with a pack of 5 or 6 wheelers and blocked wind when it was my turn, but I was often given a mulligan, especially with my bigger teammates or competitors I knew. Oh, I went as hard as I could when it was my turn but tucked into my chair, not only did I block virtually no wind for the pack behind me, but the wind forced me into a slower pace. It was better if I stayed at the back, especially if they felt I would eventually drop off the pace. It all depended upon the circumstances, but you took your turn otherwise.

But in England during that year's marathon, a male racer entered for the sole purpose of blocking the wind for his female teammate for the entire marathon. And as it turned out the number one female marathoner was wheeling by herself and leading the race until she was caught near the finish line by this tandem. It wasn't long before the rules were amended to prevent this show of poor sportsmanship from happening again.

Chapter 21: On the Road

It was back in 1980 when I moved into my one-bedroom apartment in the David B. Archer Co-op with Mr. Spock on the Esplanade, and when Bev and I got married in '85, we moved into a 2-bedroom on another floor. Now we had begun to think about a move out of the city. My parents had a different cottage in the Kawartha's, and we went there a lot on weekends so we could visit, and I could do some fishing. Driving to Buckhorn from downtown Toronto was a long process and the 401 Highway was always jam-packed coming home on a Sunday. As well, the dynamics of the city core had changed over the years, and with new developments going up all around us, and with the influx of so many more people, we decided it was time to move.

We got ourselves a real estate agent and began travelling all around the eastern outskirts of Toronto looking for the right place. The biggest obstacle being the definition of accessible. If we had gotten a dollar, for every time our agent took us to a place with stairs, or some other obvious barrier, we could have gone out to a fancy restaurant for dinner. Why the concept of "wheelchair accessible" didn't sink in, I'll never know, but we were reaching the end of our rope.

At the same time as we were looking, Gino was itching to get out of the city as well. While his disability came with different problems than with what I dealt with, he did have the advantage of being able to walk with crutches, which made accessibility not as big a priority as it was for me.

Chapter 21: On the Road

We asked him if he would like to pool his resources with us and perhaps find a place big enough for the three of us. When he thought it was a good idea, we began the search again.

As Fate would have it, my brother and his wife lived in Oshawa, and they were looking to move to a different home in the same area. Dave's wife Dianne was a registered real estate agent and more importantly, she understood the concept of "accessible". It was a no-brainer that she took over the reins of finding a place for the three of us, while she looked for a new home for her and Dave.

They found a great open-house concept place than my brother liked, and we went over to check it out. But we liked it more, and eventually, after a few hours of negotiations, the deal was done.

We bought the house. Bev and I had the upstairs and Gino had the downstairs. The three of us lived there for 5 years and then we bought him out. Dianne found him another place in Oshawa close by and we're both still in the same place after all these years.

Only two events were on my calendar that year as I finally realized it was time to pack it in for good. Bittersweet in one way because I really enjoyed wheeling in the V2 and wished the technology had been developed years earlier before all the wheeling began to take its toll on my arms.

Not to mention that moving out of town presented different problems in terms of training. The road course I took out to Cherry Beach from the Esplanade for all those years was free of hazards and included a nice wheel along the Boardwalk. Now we lived in a subdivision at the bottom of a long steep hill and Variety Village was nearly an hour away on the highway instead of a 15-minute drive.

Gino and I tried to find a suitable course that we could train on and eventually we settled on a route that didn't pose many problems. But the summer passed, and we didn't enter any races.

At the end of September, we wheeled the Dofasco Ultramarathon one last time. I wanted to lower my course record and earn another great sweatshirt.

Forty ultramarathoners lined up with the two of us for the start of the 5th edition of the 50-Miler, on a course that was virtually the same as the year before. I took off right from the gun. I wanted to go out fast and post the fastest time possible. It was a good race, weather was cool, with little wind that made it more enjoyable.

The V2 made wheeling a pleasure, even at full speed. I seemed to eat up ground as the minutes ticked by. Eventually, I took off nearly an hour of my time from the last year and crossed the finish line in 5:51:52. The coveted #1 sweat top was mine once more.

Gino finished in 6:21:15, 41 seconds ahead of able-bodied ultramarathoner Les Michalek of Burlington.

A week after wheeling the 50-miler in Hamilton, I entered the Toronto/Shopper's Drug Mark International Marathon. It was a mistake on my part, and I should have stopped mid-race when my shoulder began to give me problems. But in the two dozen marathons I entered in my career, I never failed to finish, and again, I had no intentions of stopping.

So, I pushed forward and did manage to win against the few others that had entered, but my shoulder was not the same afterwards and I was forced to stop wheeling for a couple of months. By the time spring rolled around, my shoulder was still not 100%, and I held off wheeling a while longer. Eventually, the whole summer was over, and I realized my racing career had finally come to an end.

Post-Script

Retirement was not an easy thing to get through in the beginning, though. After 20 years of feeling like a "somebody", I felt reduced to being a "nobody", just another guy in a wheelchair. It would take awhile before I felt comfortable in my own skin again.

Back in the early days, when you retired, you vanished from sight. If you didn't start coaching or stay involved in some capacity, you dropped off the map.

There was no smooth transition. You just felt that you were no longer useful. You were on your own. There were no steps supplied to help you see the future without wheelchair sports. It was depressing to say the least.

It took a couple of years to finally get used to the loss of the daily routine that previously made up my day. The best part about the free time I suddenly had, was the opportunity to enjoy one of my greatest passions: fishing for largemouth bass throughout the many lakes found in the Kawarthas.

But after a half dozen years of boating and enjoying all the free time, a conversation with one of my fellow employees at War Amps in '98, started me on a run of nearly twenty years playing sledge hockey with the Markham Islanders. I was still playing with the team when COVID-19 closed all sports.

As I began to wrap up writing this book, I wanted to check on the state of wheelchair racing once the pandemic-delayed 2020 Tokyo Paralympics were over. Just to see how far we had progressed since the '92 Barcelona Games. And while I soon realized that the modern-day racing chair was an unbelievable machine to behold, I realized some of the same negative things that went on in my era, were continuing to plague the sport, years later.

Classification was, and still is a contentious subject, and it seems to have gotten worse in a couple of areas. There have always been athletes that didn't try very hard in the tests in hopes of landing in a lower class. And there have always been doctors or "classification officials", that were willing to help an athlete cheat for the glory of their country. I'm afraid that hasn't changed.

What has changed is that every disability group now wants to be a part of the Paralympic movement. As someone who was born disabled, I can see where someone with a disability would like the opportunity to compete against their peers in whatever form of competition it would take. However, I'm not too sure about, say, nationally ranked able-bodied swimmers who had a situation that prevented them from competing at the highest level in their sport, but could still swim with ease, who suddenly became an unbeaten Paralympic athlete.

And on the other hand, I read stories about athletes who are disabled, some in wheelchairs, that are deemed unclassifiable under the existing classification guidelines. How is that possible?

So, we allow almost able-bodied athletes, with the barest of disabilities, to dominate their sport without any true competition, and that's OK, but someone who is obviously disabled, is unable to be classified? What's wrong with this picture?

Another fallout to opening the door to every conceivable disability was the impact it has on the Games themselves. Few seem to remember that ALL disabled sports owe its beginnings to Sir Ludwig Guttman and the Stoke Mandeville Hospital for starting the first Paralympic Games. The operative word being paraplegic. These were games for the wheelchair athletes of the world.

Decades later we saw the amputees form their own organizations as did the blind and the athletes who had cerebral palsy. Eventually, these three groups were represented at the Paralympics, as well.

Now there are so many categories of disabled athletes that the games are getting large and expensive. Something must give. To accommodate the range of events offered for all these disabilities, it seems that some of the traditional events are being phased out and classes are being combined, with detrimental results. And most of phased out events seem to be coming from wheelchair sports.

In my day, we had 3 racing classes for quadriplegics and 4 classes for the para-athlete, and eventually all disability classes wheeled the 100 metres, all the way up to the marathon, and all distances in between.

Now there are 2 Classes for each of the quad and para-athletes, and the events offered have severely diminished as the years have gone on.

Perhaps we need to assess the current state of the Paralympics and think about the advantages that separate Paralympic Games for each of the disability groups might bring. Many people I've talked to were not in favour of the idea, feeling that all of us together on the same stage makes a bigger statement. And that might be true, but if we must continue to sacrifice the participation of one disability group to cater to another, I don't see that as progress.

An obvious advantage, from my way of thinking, is that with your own set of games, organizers would be better able to schedule events, to maximize exposure. Combining disability groups into the same event is a TV viewer's nightmare, especially in the pool.

Without an analyst to explain the difference between the disabilities and the impact it has on an individual's performance, watching someone come last by a large margin does not begin the tell the story that had just unfolded. They might have just produced a world record in their disability class, but what it evoked was sympathy. Not what we're trying for.

One of the most glaring differences between organizing an event for each disability groups, is the difference in mobility. Staging a large wheelchair event requires accessible accommodations, washrooms, even the venue itself to be wheelchair friendly. Without those barriers to contend with, I would think that other disability groups would have a wider range of options when preparing to host their Games, and a lot less expense to stage them.

From a governing body point of view, I learned that in 1989 the International Paralympic Committee was formed, with Canada's Bob Steadward as its first President, and in 1997 the Stoke Mandeville Games were changed to the World Wheelchair Games.

Then in 2005, the competition was called the World Wheelchair and Amputee Games, and eventually, in 2009 the games were then referred to as the International Wheelchair and Amputee Sports World Games (IWAS World Games).

One bone of contention I heard frequently while doing research for this book, was that qualifying standards for the Paralympics were too high.

So, let's be clear, not everyone wants to be a full-time racer. In the beginning kids only want to wheel and have a good time. Getting fit is a by-product. The junior ranks should have no set goals to reach, other than improving their performance as a means of gaining a better level of fitness and good health. Any athlete could choose to train to achieve higher goals if they wished to.

Moving from your provincial games, to competing at the nationals takes hours of hard work. But making the Paralympic standards so hard to reach, it limits the number of participants in any given event. That in part justified the rationale of eliminating events, due to the low number of athletes in the field.

Another problem is the high cost of the ultra-modern racing chair, making it difficult for parents to afford thousands of dollars for a chair that may not fit their child in a year or so. However, I'm afraid that the cost of a racing chair is always going to be expensive, regardless, since the amount of time and money that goes into the modern racer cannot help but make it a costly piece of equipment.

For the new racing chair is a work of art. If the chairs of the late '80s replaced the *shopping carts* we used in the beginning, the new machines have done that to our old 4-wheel chairs. The advancements have been unbelievable.

From a technical standpoint, bare spoked rear wheels are mostly outdated. At first, the spokes were covered in thin plastic to make them more aerodynamic, but eventually they were replaced by real carbon fibre wheels that sported three or four large spokes. In time solid carbon fibre disc wheels appeared, which a lot of the racers around the world now use.

The hand-rims have gone through some changes as well. Once everyone began to literally punch the rims instead of gripping, the push-rims were made thinner and closer to the disc wheels. With a distinct camber on the wheels, it made it easier to apply pressure to the rims without losing grip.

This pushing style also generated the advancement of the racing glove. No longer did athletes make their own; specially made gloves to suit the new style of propulsion have been invented, and most athletes in the world now use a variation of these gloves to apply pressure to the rims and rear wheels.

The new frames are now mostly all carbon fibre or hi-strength aluminum and look a lot like the frame I had hoped to wheel in decades ago. These sleek machines come equipped with a modern compensator and steering handles.

One notable difference is the seating position. Once we realized that any extra body movement was counter productive, the bucket became an extremely tight fit. As well, a lot of attention was put towards being as aerodynamic as possible, especially on the road where top end speed had been increasing steadily.

The modern racers now have two choices of frames. Some athletes wheel with their legs tucked underneath the bucket, with a section of material that fits under the chair and allows the wind to pass underneath without impacting the chair's speed.

Other athletes that are amputees or racers that can bend their legs, race in what is know as a "kneeler". The athlete kneels on their legs and their lower body is completely encased in the bucket. Whether that makes your legs go to sleep, probably depends upon each individual athlete level of circulation, but it doesn't look comfortable.

But regardless of the style of racer they wheel in, the body position is such now, that you lay your chest on your bent knees, with the only movement being the arms, which pound down on the rims, and obtain full extension before the stroke is repeated.

And all this technology costs money. Many of the world-class racers have monetary sponsors, which allows them to race all over the world in the best equipment available. Just recently, a few racers have sponsors that are aligned with motorcar racing and have developed state-of-the-art machines, propelling these athletes to constant success.

The price of a super chair ranges from almost five thousand dollars and up to the thirty thousand for the Honda-built racer that debuted in Tokyo. Certainly, out of the range of your regular athlete that pays his own way and finances his own chair.

But the "regular" racing chair still costs in the $4,000 range, which makes it extremely difficult for parents to come up with that type of money, especially if the individual just wants the exercise and is not planning to make this his career.

There was one fact I found out while writing this book that kind of surprised me, and that was the fact that disabled athletes from some countries are now paid for winning medals. I knew that able-bodied athletes got some form of compensation, but I didn't realize that disabled athletes were receiving money as well. And I don't mean a little money. While this form of reward is not yet available in Canada, it is a growing trend.

I do see a problem when an athlete from a country that has a dubious record of how they treat their disabled citizens, receives so much compensation that they are elevated to such a status that they are removed from the daily struggles that their fellow disabled countrymen must contend with. I'm not sure that's progress either.

Another one of the biggest reasons that wheelchair racing has seen declining numbers, was the invention of the handcycle, a three-wheeled low-slung machine that the athletes lie in, with just their head elevated and using a setup like a bicycle to propel the machine forward.

Using the two-handed mechanical crank, it enabled an individual to travel much longer distances with a lot less effort. The regular racing chair requires considerable effort to go fast, and technique is critical. In a handcycle, all you do is hold the handles and crank.

Once they became popular, and races were eventually offered, many athletes who might have gotten into a racing chair, now have an alternative to getting in shape, or embarking on an actual racing career in a hand-cycle.

Another unfortunate situation is the lack of coaching and funding at the lower levels of the sport. In some countries, the elite seem to be the focus of the sports organization's finances, with little regard for the rest of the athletes.

Post-Script

I hear too often that the last crop of retired world class racers have not continued their involvement in wheelchair racing. World class coaching is certainly needed if a country's success is to be continued, but there doesn't seem to be enough interest or finances to allow individuals to pursue coaching once their own racing career was over.

Wheelchair marathons have been hit hard as well. Many marathons have dropped the wheelchair division altogether. Some cities have enacted by-laws to prevent all but runners to enter a road race.

Toronto has not had a wheelchair division for so many years, I was unable to find any records that far back. I'd hate to think I was the last wheeler to tackle the streets of Toronto.

Detroit no longer starts in Windsor anymore either. Too many logistics to overcome. Borders around the world are no longer so easy to cross over and back.

Big name marathons in the States have had numbers drop from dozens and dozens of wheelers to just a handful. However, there are wheelchair marathons around the world with significant monetary rewards still being contested.

Five of the biggest wheelchair marathons are grouped together and are known as the World Marathon Majors.

They are comprised of the Tokyo, Boston, London, Chicago and New York marathons. Normally Boston, London and Tokyo are traditionally run in the spring, while Chicago and New York are scheduled for the fall. However, the pandemic has changed the schedule in the last couple of years and things are still not back to normal.

At this moment in time, the most successful male wheelchair racer is Switzerland's Marcel Hug, who wheels in a multi-thousand-dollar racing chair, and who not only won multiple gold at the Tokyo Paralympics, including the marathon, but is virtually unbeatable out on the road. His main competition is America's Daniel Romanchuk and Canada's Brent Lakatos, winner of 4 Paralympic silver medals in Tokyo. Just recently, Hug broke the 22-year-old marathon world record that was held by his countryman Hans Frei, in winning the Tokyo marathon in the incredible time of 1:13:17.

While the new racers have certainly helped lower the world records to times that us veterans never dreamed could be possible, the future of wheelchair racing is up in the air. With more and more athletes using hand-cycles to race in, our sport is now called push-rim racing and seems to have it's future resting on the road circuit as more and more obstacles present themselves at the Paralympic level.

Regardless of the future state of wheelchair racing, it was certainly a privilege and honour to represent my country through the 21 years that I competed. The chance to travel around the world, wearing Canada's colours helped mold me into the confident person I am right now, and that was accomplished as a member of Canada's Paralympic Team.

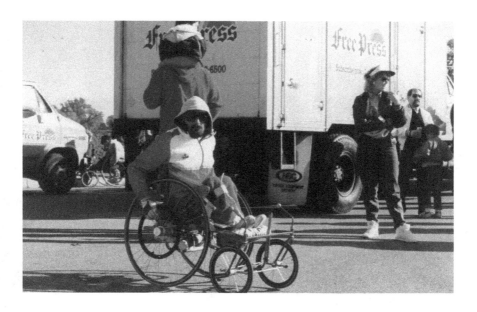

Getting ready for the 1986 Detroit Free Press Marathon

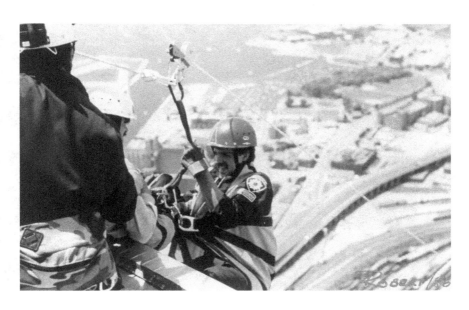

Toronto CN Tower jump -Canada Day July 1, 1986

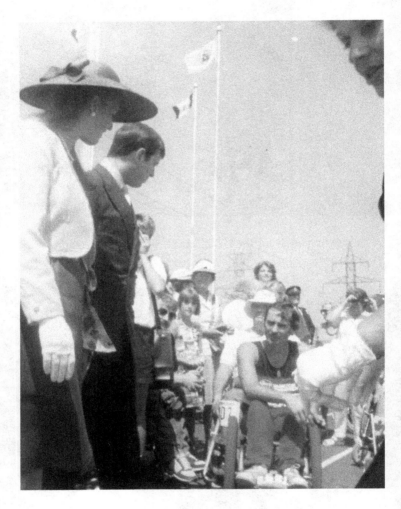

Chatting with the Royals prior to my slalom demonstration at the 1987 Ontario Games

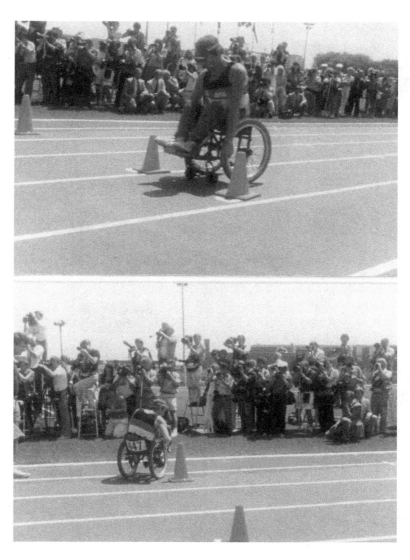

a throng of photographers watch the Royals watching my slalom demo

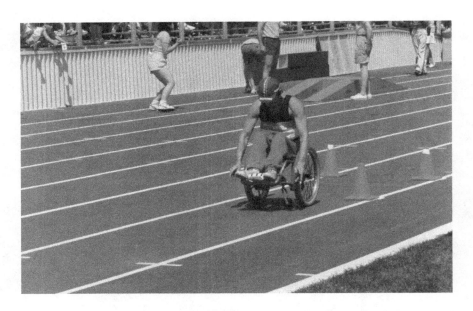

1987 Provincials - slalom final

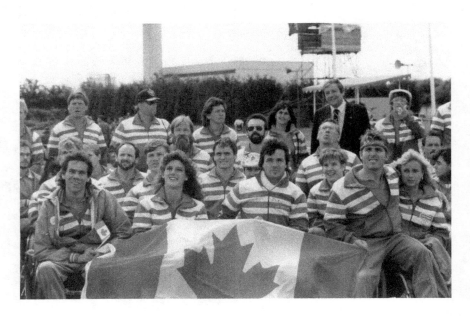

opening ceremonies for the 1987 World Championships in Stoke Mandeville England

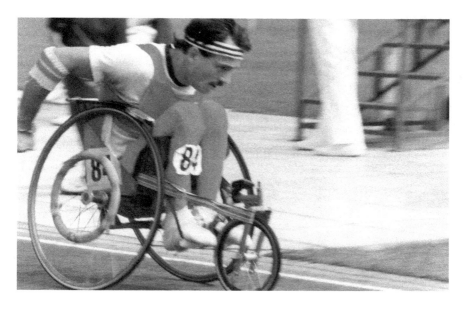

Canada's Paul Clark, inventor of the world's first 3-wheel racing chair, heading for gold during the 1987 World Championships in England

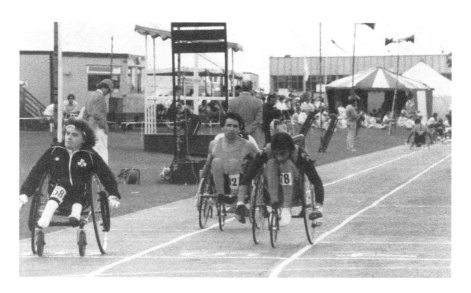

Canada's super quads Bob Ellery (82) and Clayton Gerein (78) warming up during the 1987 World Championships

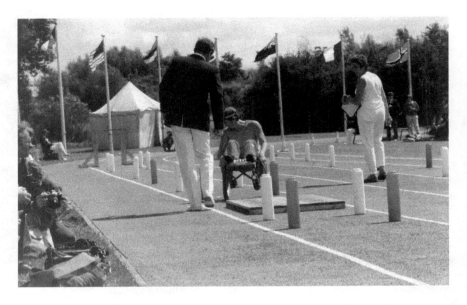

in the lead during round one of the Class 3 slalom event during the 1987 World Championships

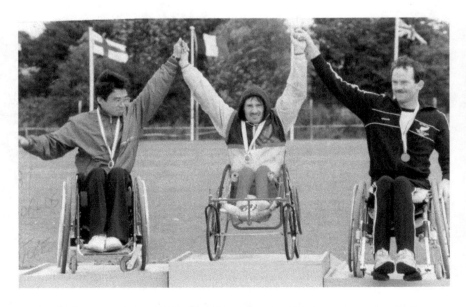

Sitting on top of the podium for the slalom medal presentation ceremony during the 1987 World Championships

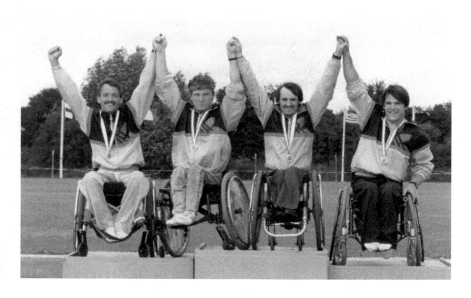

1987 4 x 400 relay medal presentation (l-r) Paul Clark - Chris Daw - Chris Stoddart - Ron Robillard

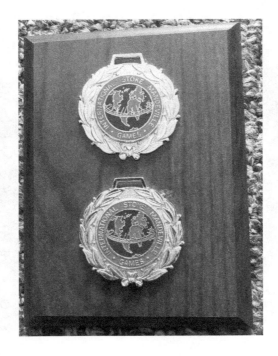

my gold medals from winning the Class 3 slalom and as a member of the 4 x 400 metre relay team during the 1987 World Championships

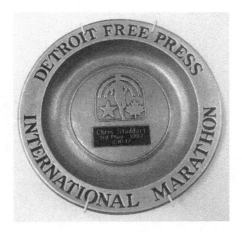

pewter plate from the 1987 Detroit Free Press marathon

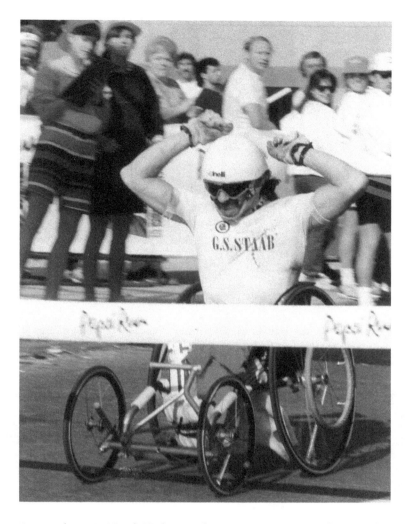

winning the 1989 North York Marathon in my new Top End racing chair

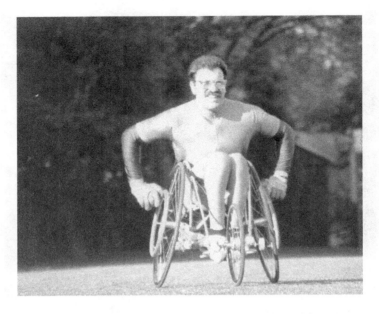

CP racer Gino Vendetti, silver medal winner in the 200 and 400 metres at the 1988 Seoul Paralympics, warming up in the new V2 racer in the spring of 1991.

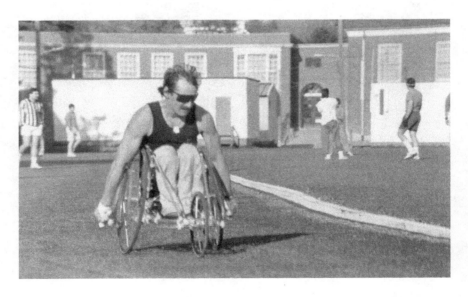

first time in my new Andre Viger V2 racing chair in the spring of 1990

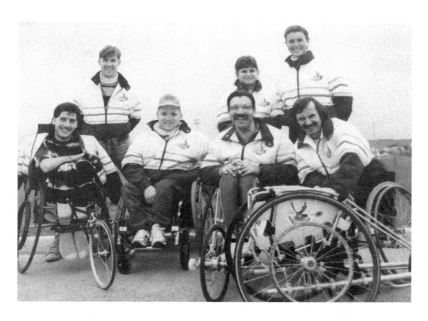

Phoenix Track Club - Randy Marsh - Laura Misciagna - Kelly McLeod in back and Martin Larocque - Keith Brettell - Gino Vendetti and Chris Stoddart in front

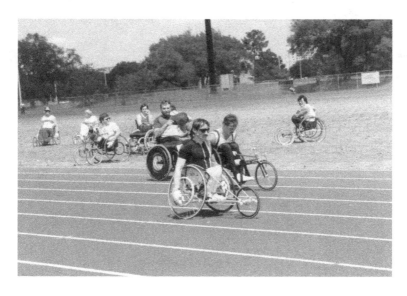

Warming up with American legend George Murray during the 1991 Tampa Florida Sunshine Games

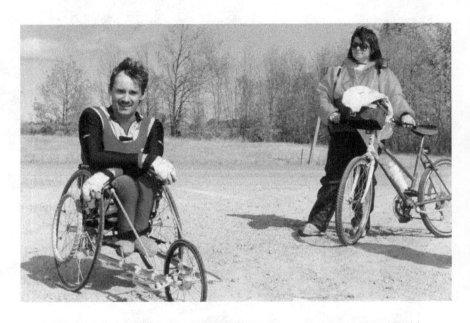

After 20 years of racing, Bev and I wait for the start of the Dofasco Golden Horseshoe 50-miler, my last big race.

Canadian Paralympic Wheelchair Track Medalists

1968 Tel Aviv, Israel

Gord Paterson (Class A) Gold (60 Metre)

Duncan Wilson (Class B) Gold (60 Metre)

Walter Dann (Class C) Silver (60 Metre)

Oren Bourne (Class B) Bronze (Slalom)

Hilda Binns (Class B) Gold (60 Metre) Silver (Slalom)

1972 Heidelberg, West Germany

Bob Simpson (Class 5) Gold (100 Metre)

Doug Bovee (Class 1A) Gold (Slalom) Silver (60 Metre)

Frank Henderson / Walter Dann / Gene Reimer / Bob Simpson (Class 2-5) Silver (4 X 60 Metre Relay)

Hilda Binns (Class 3) Silver (60 Metre) (Slalom)

Sharon Long (Class 1B) Bronze (Slalom)

1976 Toronto Canada

Pete Colistro (Class 5) Gold (800 Metre) Silver (1500 Metre)

Chris Stoddart (Class 4) Bronze (800 Metre) (Slalom)

Ed Batt (Class 1A) Bronze (Slalom)

Joanne McDonald (Classss 5) Silver (Slalom)

1980 Arnhem, Netherlands

Ed Batt (1A) Bronze (Slalom)

Gary Birch (Class 1A) Silver (60 Metre)

Mel Fitzgerald (Class 5) Gold (800 Metre) (1500 Metre) Silver (100 Metre)

Rick Hansen (Class 4) Gold (800 Metre) Silver (1500 Metre)

Ron Minor (Class 4) Bronze (Slalom)

Andre Viger / Ron Minor / Rick Hansen / Mel Fitzgerald (Class 2-5) Bronze (4x100 Metre Relay)

Pam Frazee (Class 3) Bronze (400 Metre)

Joanne McDonald (Class 5) Gold (Slalom)

1984 Stoke Mandeville, England

Paul Clark (Class 2) Gold (800 Metre) Silver (200 – 400 – 1500 - 5,000 Metre - Marathon)

Mel Fitzgerald (Class 5) Gold (Marathon) Silver (1500 - 5,000 Metre) Bronze (800 Metre)

Terry Gehlert (1B) Bronze (100 Metre)

Rick Hansen (Class 4) Gold (Marathon) (1500 Metre) Silver (5,000 Metre)

Ron Minor (Class 4) Gold (200 – 400 – 800 Metre) Bronze (Marathon – 100 Metre Metre)

Ross Sampson (Class 3) Bronze (Marathon)

Chris Stoddart (Class 3) Silver (Slalom)

Andre Viger (Class 3) Gold (Marathon) Bronze (1500 Metre)

Paul Clark / Ron Minor / Rick Hansen / Mel Fitzgerald (Class 2-5) Silver (4x100 Relay) (4x200 Relay) (4x400 Relay)

Martha Gustafson (Class 1A) Gold (100 – 200 – 400 – 800 Metre)

Angela Ieriti (Class 5) Gold (800 – 1500 – 5,000 Metre) Silver (200 – 400 Metre)

Debbie Kostelyk (Class 3) Gold (100 – 400 Metre) Silver (200 Metre)

Diane Rakieki (Class 4) Silver (800 Metre)

Tham Simpson (Class 1C) Gold (Slalom - 100 – 200 – 400 – 800 Metre)

Judy Zelman (Class 1C) Bronze (200 – 400 Metre)

1988 Seoul, Korea

Jeff Adams (Class 5/6) Bronze (800 – 1500 Metre)

Andre Beaudoin (Class 1C) Gold (200 Metre) Silver (100 – 400 Metre) Bronze (800 Metre)

Paul Clark (Class 2) Gold (800 Metre) Silver (Marathon – 1500 Metre)

Clayton Gerein (Class 1B) Gold (400 – 800 – 5,000 Metre) Silver (1500 Metre) Bronze (Marathon)

Marc Quessy (Class 2) Gold (Marathon) Silver (100 Metre)

Serge Raymond (Class 1B) Gold (Marathon – 200 – 1500 Metre)

Daryl Stubel (Class 1B) Silver (400 Metre)

Andre Viger (Class 3) Gold (Marathon) Silver (10,000 Metre) Bronze (5,000 Metre)

Ted Vince (Class 5/6) Bronze (Marathon – 400 Metre)

Dan Westley (Amp) Gold (100 – 800 Metre) Silver (200 – 400 – 1500 – 5,000 Metre)

Debbie Kostelyk (Class 3) Silver (100 Metre)

1992 Barcelona, Spain

Jeff Adams (Class Tw4) Silver (800 Metre)

Andre Viger (Class Tw3) Gold (10,000 Metre)

Andre Beaudoin (Class Tw2) Silver (100 Metre) Bronze (200 Metre)

Clayton Gerein (Class Tw2) Gold (Marathon – 5,000 Metre) Bronze (800 – 1500 Metre)

Luke Gingras (Class Tw3) Bronze (200 – 800 Metre)

Marc Quessy (Class Tw3) Silver (200 – 400 Metre)

Richard Reelie (Class Tw2) Gold (400 – 800 Metre) Silver (200 – 1500 Metre)

James Baker / Marc Quessey / Andre Viger / Dan Westley (Tw 3-4) Silver (4x100 Metre Relay)

Luke Gingras / Marc Quessey / Andre Viger / Jeff Adams (Tw 3-4) Silver (4x400 Metre Relay)

Colette Bourgonje (Class Tw3) Bronze (100 – 800 Metre)

Kristine Harden (Class Tw2) Gold (400 – 800 Metre) Silver (200 Metre)

Chantal Peticlerc (Class Tw4) Bronze (200 – 800 Metre)

1996 Atlanta, Georgia

Jeff Adams (Class T53) Gold (800 Metre) Silver (400 Metre)

Andre Beaudoin (Class T51) Silver (100 Metre) Bronze (400 Metre)

Dean Bergeron (Class T51) Gold (200 Metre) Silver (400 – 800 – 1500 Metre) Bronze (100 Metre)

Clayton Gerein (Class T51) Gold (5,000 Metre) Silver (Marathon) Bronze (1500 Metre)

Marc Quessey (Class T52) Bronze (800 Metre)

Brent McMahon (Class T51) Gold (Marathon)

Colin Mathieson / Carl Marquis / Marc Quessey / Jeff Adams
(Class T52-T53) Bronze (4 X 400 Metre Relay)

Colette Bourgonje (Class T52) Bronze (100 – 200 Metre)

Chantal Peticlerc (Class T53) Gold (100 – 200 Metre)
Silver (400 – 800 – 1500 Metre)

2000 Sydney, Australia

Jeff Adams (Class T54) Gold (800 – 1500 Metre) Silver (400 Metre)
Bronze (5,000 Metre)

Andre Beaudoin (Class T52) Silver (200 Metre) Bronze (100 Metre)

Clayton Gerein (Class T52) Gold (Marathon)

Dean Bergeron (Class T52) Bronze (200 – 400 Metre)

Richard Reelie (Class T52) Silver (800 – 1500 Metre)

Barry Patriquin / Mathieu Blanchette / Mathieu Parent / Jeff Adams
(Class 51-53) Bronze (4 X 100 Metre Relay)

Lisa Franks (Class T52) Gold (200 – 400 – 800 – 1500 Metre)
Silver (100 Metre)

Chantal Peticlerc (Class T54) Gold (200 – 800 Metre)
Silver (100 – 400 Metre)

2004 Athens, Greece

Jeff Adams (Class T54) Bronze (400 Metre)

Andre Beaudoin (Class T52) Gold (200 Metre) Silver (400 Metre)
Bronze (100 Metre)

Dean Bergeron (Class T52) Bronze (800 Metre)

Clayton Gerein (Class T52) Bronze (Marathon)

Kelly Smith (Class T54) Silver (Marathon)

Lisa Franks (Class T52) Gold (200 – 400 Metre)

Jessica Matassa (Class T54) Bronze (800 Metre)

Chantal Peticlerc (Class T54) Gold (100 – 200 – 400 – 800 – 1500 Metre)

Diane Roy (Class T54) Bronze (400 – 1500 Metre)

2008 Beijing, China

Andre Beaudoin (Class T52) Bronze (100 Metre)

Dean Bergeron (Class T52) Gold (100 – 200 Metre) Bronze (400 Metre)

Hanna Duff (Class T53) Bronze (100 Metre)

Chantal Peticlerc (Class T54) Gold (100 – 200 – 400 – 800 – 1500 Metre)

Diane Roy (Class T54) Silver (5,000 Metre) Bronze (400 – 800 Metre)

Michelle Stilwell (Class T52) Gold (100 – 200 Metre)

2012 London, England

Brent Lakatos (Class T53) Silver (200 – 400 – 800 Metre)

Michelle Stilwell (Class T52) Gold (200 Metre) Silver (100 Metre)

2016 Rio De Janeiro, Brazil

Brent Lakatos (Class T53) Gold (100 Metre) Silver (400 Metre) Bronze (800 Metre)

Tristan Smyth / Curtis Thom / Alexandre Dupont / Brent Lakatos) Bronze (4 X 400 Metre Relay)

Michelle Stilwell (Class T52) Gold (100 – 400 Metre)

2020 Tokyo, Japan

Brent Lakatos (Class T53) Silver (100 – 400 – 800 – 5,000 Metre)

CPSIA information can be obtained
at www.ICGtesting.com
Printed in the USA
BVHW062310070123
655774BV00004B/7